SUPERHAIR

SUPERHAIR

THE DOCTOR'S BOOK OF BEAUTIFUL HAIR

●

Jonathan Zizmor, M.D. and John Foreman

Published by
Berkley Publishing Corporation

Distributed by
G.P. Putnam's Sons, New York

SBN: 399-12005-X

Library of Congress Cataloging in Publication Data

Zizmore, Jonathan.
    Superhair : the doctor's book of beautiful hair.

    Includes index.
    1. Hair—Care and hygiene. I. Foreman, John,
1945- joint author. II. Title.
RL91.Z55   1978   646.7'24   77-22817

PRINTED IN THE UNITED STATES OF AMERICA

Contents

Part III. Medical Help for Your Hair—
Common Problems and Cures

Part IV. Why Hair Falls Out—
and What You Can Do About It

Part V. What You Can Learn from Your Hair

Preface

Beautiful hair is crucial to good looks. But how many of us *really* know what's best for our hair? As long as advertising copywriters and enthusiastic salespeople remain the prime source of information about hair, the American public will continue to throw away millions of dollars on esoteric conditioners, exotic shampoos, unorthodox grooming aids, jazzy appliances, weird coloring agents, thickeners, and salon treatments of every description, many of which have no value at all.

This book, written by a doctor and filled with medically correct advice, is designed to correct all this misinformation. The author's aim is to teach the reader how hair grows and what can—and cannot—be done to and for it. To illustrate the present level of public misunderstanding, consider the following statements:

1. Daily shampooing is bad for the hair.
2. Hair yanked out by the roots never grows back.
3. Scalp massage stimulates hair growth.
4. Brushing a hundred strokes a day is good for your hair.

5. Ultraviolet-light exposure accelerates hair growth.
6. Special vitamin supplements will make the hair shine.

The above statements are all false. And it's a depressing fact that most people who buy hair products operate on these and other similar false assumptions.

So what is the best thing to do with hair that is too dry, too thin, or too dull? And what about people with unruly mops or with the famous frizzies?

At present, professional, medically oriented advice about hair is practically nonexistent. People with poor hair are usually either too embarrassed or too intimidated to take their complaint to a busy family doctor dermatologist. So they wind up "learning" all sorts of bogus "secrets" from fashionable "hair-treatment salons" or from the proponents of mad theories involving strange herbs, diets, rays—and worse.

The purpose of this book is twofold. First, we'll demythologize hair and reveal the fascinating realities of its true physical nature. You'll learn how and why hair grows, what makes it flourish, how it is harmed, and genuinely effective ways to restore reversible damage. Second, within these pages you'll find invaluable cosmetic information. The most frequently asked hair-care questions will be answered individually and informatively, and there's lots of advice on products, too. I've restricted myself to commonsense recommendations in order to give you a guide as useful in the shower as in the beauty parlor.

There are also readable and illuminating sections on medical problems such as dandruff, psoriasis, and fungal infections. There's news on the latest methods of hair replacement. Plus a unique do-it-yourself home analysis that will enable you to profile your own hair, discover its strengths and weaknesses, analyze the cause of conditions like dullness, split ends, or hair loss, and even predict your hair's own future.

Pay special attention to my advice on hair products. After

reading the descriptions of what does—and does not—affect hair, you'll be immunized against hair quackery. Armed with a knowledge of simple medical truths, you'll be able to select products that will most effectively treat your specific hair problem.

The book is divided into six sections: Part I, Making the Most of Your Own Hair; Part II, Hair Help from Professionals; Part III, Medical Help for Your Hair—Common Problems and Cures; Part IV, Why Hair Falls Out—and What You Can Do About It; Part V, What You Can Learn from Your Hair; Part VI, Formulary. I've tried to include within these pages answers to hair questions I've been asked repeatedly in many years of teaching and practicing dermatology. I've also tried to make the book enjoyable to read and easy to use. I hope it will save you money and help you look your best.

Part I
Making the Most of Your Own Hair

1

Why Hair Grows

The first—and most important—thing to understand about hair is its relation to its roots. Many people wrongly think that if they yank hard on their hair, they'll drag out a subsurface structure, without which new hair won't grow. Well, relax; hair doesn't have roots the way trees or grass does. You *can't* yank out hair roots by yanking out hair.

Each hair on your head (and body) is a completely lifeless protein structure. It is produced beneath the skin surface by a *follicle*, which is simply one of the body's many structures. Follicles are little bulbous structures buried deeply and safely in the lower layers of the skin. Just as your liver produces bile and your stomach produces digestive juices, so your follicles produce *keratin*, the protein substance commonly called *hair*.

Each hair is detachable from its follicle. In fact, all hairs naturally fall out in regular cycles, after which the follicles grow replacements. If you yank a hair out before its normal shed cycle has arrived, you will actually stimulate new growth. That's why women seeking Jean Harlow eyebrows should shave their brows, not pluck them.

People with rich, full heads of hair do not have *more* hair follicles than Yul Brynner, but they do have better genetically inherited hormones that control both the quality and the quantity of hair on the head and body. Everybody has about 100,000 follicles on the scalp, but the people with especially thick, luxuriant hair may also have the following: 1) low levels of follicle-shriveling androgenic (male) hormones, and/or 2) follicles that are resistant to the effects of androgenic hormones by virtue of genetic inheritance, and/or 3) good levels of estrogenic (female) hormones that naturally counter the androgens, and/or 4) long and sustained growth cycles. Conclusion: The essential quality of your hair is predetermined by your genes. You can't change what nature gave you, but you *can* cosmetically improve the hair you were born with. But more on this later.

THE CYCLES OF HAIR GROWTH

Now we come to the natural—and, frankly, mysterious—cycles that govern the growth of all human and animal hair. Like many other natural phenomena, these cycles can be much better described than explained. Basically, every follicle produces a hair according to a three-part growth-and-shed cycle. This cycle continuously repeats itself until at some unpredictable point in the life of each follicle, growth permanently stops. During its lifetime each follicle undergoes the cycle independent of every other. If the growth and shed phases occurred simultaneously on the whole scalp, we'd all go bald periodically. Instead, at any given time a certain amount of hair is growing on our heads.

Hair follicles have amazing properties. For one thing, they are among the most rapidly metabolizing organs in the human body. Think of them as miniature gas-swilling limousines, gobbling a disproportionate amount of nutrients from the bloodstream. For just this reason, the blood-supply system in the human scalp is extremely highly developed, which also explains why head wounds bleed especially heavily.

Limousines produce horsepower as follicles produce keratin: Feed the limousine low-test gas, and it will cough and sputter; deprive your bloodstream of essential proteins or calories due to an unbalanced and insufficient diet, and your follicles won't produce good keratin.

Human bodies grow two types of hair: *terminal,* which grows on the head, eyebrows, pubis, and underarms, and *villous,* the peach fuzz on arms, cheeks, and bodies. Although these two kinds of hair substantially differ, the same follicles are capable of growing either one. This is why peach fuzz on adolescent cheeks turns to tough beards, why bald men sometimes have fuzzy scalps, and why leg hairs may become increasingly tough and unsightly as the body matures.

More interesting facts about follicles: Certain animals, like deer, can and do grow new follicles all the time. Humans, however, have a finite number, which must last them all their lives. Fortunately, follicles never die, although as age advances, many cease to produce hair, shrinking instead and hanging in a sort of suspended animation while a certain amount is falling out. Even on the baldest heads the follicles aren't dead, only dormant, and the current medical explanation for baldness is that accumulations of androgenic hormones in the bloodstream somehow permanently interrupt the continuity of the three-part growth-and-shed cycle.

The first phase of the three-part cycle, called the *anagen phase,* is a period of extremely rapid keratin production. The bulblike follicle expands and extends deeper into the nourishing network of subsurface blood vessels, but despite the rapid metabolic activity, hair will seem to grow slowly. The

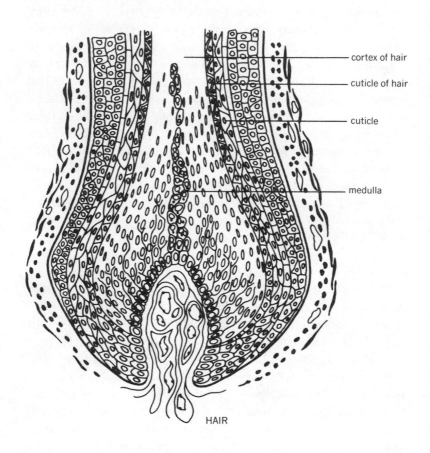

1) A single strand of hair, as it would appear if viewed through a microscope.

average rate of growth of a human hair for the duration of the anagen phase is only about a third of a millimeter per day. If you take a 100-millimeter cigarette, divide it by 100, then divide that hundredth into thirds, each third would represent the amount of daily hair growth during the anagen phase.

The hair that's pushed out of the anagen follicle looks almost like a little pole with three layers and a detachable base thrust into the follicle. The outer layer is called the *cuticle* (although it bears no relation to fingernail cuticles); beneath the cuticle is a softer structure called the *cortex;* and at the center of the pole is a core called the *medulla.* Even though the cuticle, cortex, and medulla have structural differences, they are all made of keratin.

We should note here that grooming hair means keeping the hair cuticles in good condition. When the hard protective outer cuticle is dried out or worn off by too much washing, too-strong shampoo, too much sunlight, or too much blow drying, the softer cortex and medulla become vulnerable, and when these structures fray, as they will without the cuticle to protect them, the result is split ends, dullness, and lack of control.

As the anagen phase progresses, this hardened three-layered structure of keratin continues to be pushed up out of the follicle opening and past the scalp surface. Just below the surface of the scalp a tiny oil gland that channels into the follicle provides lubrication for the newly emerging hair.

The length of each hair follicle's anagen phase varies significantly from one person to another, usually lasting somewhere between two and six years.

Although human hair-growth phases are staggered in a mosaic pattern, there are some animals whose follicles go through the growth and shed phases simultaneously. They

would lose their hair the way a snake sheds its skin were it
not for the convenient fact that their anagen phase is longer
than their expected life-span. Merino sheep fall into this
category, as do rats, mice, and French poodles.

For us humans, anagen-phase hair continues to be pushed
up out of the follicles just like toothpaste out of a tube. The
exact length of this phase is affected by genetics and/or age:
A follicle's anagen phase is longer for a teenager than for a
forty-year-old. But, inevitably, anagen must stop and the next
phase must begin.

The *catagen*, or transitional, *phase* of the growth cycle is
brief, sometimes lasting only a matter of weeks. During this
period the catagen follicle winds down its rapid metabolism,
wrinkles, contracts, and ceases the production of keratin.
Incidentally, scalp massages to increase blood flow on the
scalp are ineffective in reversing this natural phase of follicle
shrinkage. Catagen shrinkage is a natural pact of the growth-
and-shed cycle, and there's no way to stop it.

The final phase of the growth-and-shed cycle, called the
telogen phase, occurs when the follicle stops shrinking. This
is a period of rest and suspended animation in which the hair
does not immediately fall out but, rather, sits in the now
fully contracted follicle bulb. The typical length of the
telogen phase is around three months, during which the hair
will rest in the follicle until it's physically dislodged by
brushing or washing. At any given time you can normally
expect about 15 percent of your follicles to be in either the
catagen or the telogen phase, and the other 85 percent will
be in anagen, actively growing hair.

What precipitates the end of anagen and the onset of the
transitional and shed phases? Although not much is medically
proved, it has been observed that childbirth and similar
shocks to the total physical system commonly cause a
substantial loss of hair called *telogen effluvium.* Actually, this

is a positive sign, since the falling hair is usually being pushed out by new anagen growth.

Any major shock—psychological or physical—can terminate anagen and bring on telogen in a substantial number of follicles. Starting to take birth-control pills or discontinuing them can do it, as can extremely stressful emotional situations, illnesses and accidents. But even in the absence of a trauma each follicle will naturally reach a point where it terminates anagen activity, much the way a tree simply stops growing at a certain point in the fall.

Scientists understand the tree much better than the hair follicle, but it is interesting to note that follicles shed keratin when trees shed leaves—in the fall. And if a person were to move from America to Australia, it may be only a short time before his or her follicle adjusted to the reversed seasons and began to shed hair when autumn occurred down there.

Falling hair is natural, and now I will make a statement which I know will be surprising: Whenever you seem to be losing a sudden and unnatural amount of hair, you should be *encouraged*. In nine cases out of ten it means that telogen follicles, whose hairs have *not* been growing but only resting in contracted follicles, have reverted to the anagen phase of production, in which the new growth is pushing out the lame-duck telogen hair. Permanent and irreversible hair loss advances much more gradually and is usually unnoticeable until it's well advanced.

I have met many people who cut down on shampooing and brushing in order to stop their hair from falling out. They see clumps of hairs trapped on the brush or bunched in the shower drain, and they panic. Remember, it is normal to lose anywhere from 70 to 200 hairs *every day*. Cutting down on shampooing means only that when you do shampoo, even more loose hairs will collect in the shower drain, including

many that have become detached since the last shampoo or
brushing.

Let me stress again that telogen hairs fall out as a result of
normal and natural growth cycles; average or even excessive
washing and brushing simply do not cause permanent hair
loss. Telogen hairs are doomed, for they cannot stay on the
scalp for more than a few months without the support of an
active anagen follicle. Fortunately, the average telogen hair
withstands numerous normal shampooings and brushings.

The actual falling out of telogen hair is usually enough to
stimulate the follicle and flip it back into the anagen phase.
This is the real context in which daily hair loss should be
viewed. Of course your hair, like the rest of you, has good
days and bad days. Stressful days might result in more than
average shedding, but it all equals out, since the rate of
telogen effluvium is normally constant.

I'm going to deal much more specifically with the problem
of permanent hair loss in another chapter. At this point I
want simply to state again that abundant hair is a matter of
genetic good luck. There are really two independent systems
at work here: One is the normal growth-and-shed cycle that
governs follicle activity; the other has to do with each
follicle's capacity to continue the cycle, which is thought to
be determined by hormones in the bloodstream.

Very little can be done to alter your genetic makeup. As
for your hair, it's a matter of protecting and making the most
of what you've got. Remember that massaging the scalp
doesn't do anything and that dispensing with shampooing
won't stop hair loss, but it will make your hair look dirty.

Hair grows from within. You can put anything you want
on your scalp, but it won't affect the growth rate, retard the
loss rate, or improve the quality of the hair shaft itself. There
is actually a membrane barrier between the epidermis layer
of the skin and the dermis that lies below, which effectively

protects the follicles in the dermis from substances on the epidermis. This protective membrane makes it difficult to nourish the hair follicle from above, a fact that underscores the importance of a good diet. Plenty of creams and lotions can make your hair look better *temporarily*, but what you've got is what you've got.

2

Types of Hair and
Typical Hair Problems

The golden rule of hair care is "Make the most of what you've got." You can use all sorts of grooming products to enhance your hair's appearance, but you can't change your genetic heritage.

Let's first categorize your hair and identify its basic strengths and weaknesses. This requires plucking a strand and examining it closely under a strong light. Don't worry about that hair; by plucking it you've automatically flipped the follicle back into the anagen growth phase.

1. *Coarse hair.* Coarse hair is thick in diameter and strong, sometimes almost wiry. Most people consider it a blessing unless it's so tough you can't manage it. The major advantage of coarse hair is its ability to sustain lots of washing, blow drying, grooming, curling, and coloring without damage. If you're struggling to control your hairstyle, don't curse your coarse hair; be glad that you can confidently tame it with a daily shampooing and conditioning, all of which will be discussed in Chapters 3 and 4.

2. *Fine hair.* If your sample hair is narrow, limp, and lacks body, you've got fine hair. It's important to understand that fine hair is neither a problem nor a disease, but it requires cautious handling, since too much bleaching, coloring, shampooing, blow drying, brushing, and curling will make it brittle and flyaway. Despite these problems, your fine hair has a unique texture that's absolutely beautiful if you brush it delicately, avoid regular exposure to excessive heat and chemicals, and choose mild shampoos and body-building protein conditioners.

3. *Thick hair.* Next, I want you to lift your hair upward from your forehead and observe the roots. If the hairs are densely spaced on the scalp, you've got thick hair. Lucky you, because you've got lots of hair to work with. About all you'll need is a good layered cut to reduce unwieldy bulk. If your thick hair is curly, beware of short haircuts; they can be impossible to manage. If your thick hair is straight and if you want to add curl, then you'll need a heavy-duty permanent and losts of grooming aids to counter the natural drag your heavy hair exerts on the curls. The best beauty advice for people with thick hair is to choose a style that makes the most of the hair's natural degree of curliness.

4. *Thin hair.* Thin hair, which is widely spaced on the scalp, needs body-building protein conditioners to give it fullness. Thin hair generally looks best when cut in short or medium lengths, and to achieve any fullness at all, daily shampooing and conditioning are almost imperative.

You might also consider special thickeners like **Thickit** and **Pantene,** discussed in Chapter 6.

5. *Curly hair.* If your hair already has a natural curl or wave, I advise you to make every effort to take advantage of it. People pay money to get curls like yours, including the tight, kinky ones you fought against for so long. A good layered cut that encourages the natural curl is a lot more sensible than an enforced style that fights a constantly losing

battle against it. And you'll be sparing your hair the torture of daily blowouts since most curly styles require natural or lamp drying.

6. *Straight hair.* It often seems that people with the most gorgeously straight hair are always the ones who want to be curly-headed. That's human nature. But most real concerns of straight-haired people revolve around body and fullness. Again, these problems are easily treated with the protein conditioners described in Chapter 4. It's also a good idea to beware of cuts that are too long, especially if the hair is fine and/or thin, in which case a long style can make it look stringy.

7. *Normal hair.* If your hair is neither particularly coarse nor fine, thick nor thin, curly nor straight, then it's like most people's hair: normal. The normal head can easily tolerate daily shampooing and doesn't absolutely need conditioners, although they will make your hair shinier if you use them. Normal hair can be effectively dyed or bleached without noticeable damage and will profit from a supercut by a good stylist.

Clearly, hair types are *not* mutually exclusive categories. They overlap, and the various combinations are all subject to the following hair problems.

THE FIVE MOST COMMON HAIR PROBLEMS

1. *Oiliness.* If the glands attached to your hair follicles secrete too much oil, the result is lank and greasy hair. The rate of oil secretion is again a function of your hormonal makeup, but it appears that psychological stress also stimulates production of some of the same hormones that stimulate oil glands. You actually *can* calm down and so have less oily hair, although it's usually not that easy, because your rate of oil secretion is inherited; only advancing age may slow it

down. There is, however, quite a lot you can do to remove the unwanted oil quickly, thereby keeping your hair full-bodied and lustrous.

The key to treating problem oiliness is daily shampooing. Fact: The effectiveness of a shampoo's active ingredients will *decline* with repeated use. Therefore, a good antioil regimen would include three different shampoos used alternately for three successive days. Then, on the fourth day, wash the hair with ordinary bath soap. Whatever's in the shower is okay. **Neutrogena** is particularly good, since it's very pure and mildly drying. Of course, you don't want to strip the hair too completely of natural oils, so shampoo daily, but lather only once, regardless of what the instructions say.

After your daily shampoo you'll probably need a daily conditioner to ensure manageability and to impart body to thin or fine hair. Commercial conditioners are discussed in Chapter 4, but if your oily problem is especially acute and if your hair already has natural fullness, try the following home recipes. To freshly shampooed hair apply three tablespoons of apple-cider vinegar mixed with a glass of cool water, then rinse thoroughly with more cool water. The acid vinegar closes up the natural openings on the hair cuticles, gives the hair a nice sheen and strips away excessive oil. Or, to achieve a similar effect, you might try spraying freshly shampooed hair with a plant mister filled with three tablespoons of lemon juice mixed with cool water.

If you've got problem oiliness, you should definitely settle on a shorter hairstyle, which makes daily washing easier and more effective. And you might consider a sunlamp regimen. Although the reasons are not fully understood, it has been widely observed that exposure to heat tends to retard oil secretion. That's why oil-related acne improves in the summer and why many dermatologists prescribe sunlamp treatments for oily-acne sufferers. Well, the sunlamp also seems to work on the hair. Hold the lamp in your hand and expose all parts of the dried hair with an easy, sweeping motion. Your first treatment should last a half minute, after which you can work up to three minutes by daily increments of five seconds. Although this technique doesn't work for everyone, it's worth a try, especially if you already have a sunlamp. Be sure to protect your eyes and follow the manufacturer's instructions.

2. *Dryness.* In nine cases out of ten problem dryness of the hair is *self-induced* and is unrelated to dryness of the skin. It's nearly always a result of too much shampooing, blow drying, sun exposure, chemical permanents, dyes, and not enough brushing.

The best antidryness grooming oil is produced by the glands on your own scalp. To distribute that oil properly, you should brush your hair twenty-five full strokes per day. But please remember that if you go over those twenty-five strokes, you'll run the risk of inducing *traction alopecia,* a temporary hair loss caused by too-vigorous brushing. Stick to twenty-five daily strokes, and you'll be maximizing your body's organic grooming aid.

It is imperative for the dry-haired person to cut down on those processes that aggravate dryness. Coloring or curling with harsh chemicals is definitely not advised. Naturally, you have to shampoo, but do it less often, every other day, never daily. You can also make your favorite shampoo less drying if you add two tablespoons of oil to the lather. *Any* oil will do, from Mazola to olive to drugstore-counter lanolin. Try at all costs to avoid blow drying, but if you absolutely must, at least use the lowest heat setting and don't make it a daily occurrence.

Regular conditioning for dry hair is a must and you should try a hair pack in which you wrap oil-treated hair with a hot, wet towel. You'll find details on these treatments in Chapter 4.

3. *Fragility.* Fragile hair is easily broken, usually dry, and frequently worn longer than it should be. Most of the time

the cuticle has been eroded either by age, as in extra-long hair, or abuse, if your hair is the victim of too much dying, bleaching, permanenting, or blow drying.

To protect your fragile hair, you must take immediate steps to close the natural shingles of the cuticle, which are called *imbrications*. Conditioners will play a major role in this restorative program. At the same time, you should beware of agents, like shampoos, that tend to open up the cuticle. Don't stop shampooing, but switch to baby shampoo and wash as infrequently as you can, perhaps every second or third day. If you use a blower daily, cut down immediately and save heat styling for special occasions *only*. And be very careful not to overbrush or overcomb.

Most fragility problems occur at the ends of long hairs, where the cuticle is oldest and most damaged. If the cuticle has rubbed away entirely, either the hair will break off or the cortex will fray into split ends. Protein conditioners and hair packs of the sort described in Chapter 4 can temporarily glue these ends together. But the only way to really cure split ends is to cut them off.

Some women who are actually experiencing genetically determined hair loss mistakenly think their hair is breaking off because of fragility. Occasionally superhot hair dryers or oils can kill hair follicles, but steady, inexorable hair loss is almost always inherited. If you stop all abusive practices and after four months your hair doesn't get thicker, you'll know for sure that the problem isn't fragility. Genetic hair loss is fully discussed in Part IV.

4. *Dullness.* Faded color and lack of sheen are normally caused by a combination of dryness and overexposure to strong chemicals in dyes, bleaches, and permanents. If your hair has the clarity of dirty dishwater, give it a complete rest.

For a week stop everything, including shampoos, blow drying, and conditioning. After your hair's vacation, during which you might wear it pulled back or even resort to wigs, scarves, or turbans, you should attack the probable dryness problem with the conditioning suggestions in Chapter 4. If you color your hair, I'd recommend you see a professional colorist for advice. Continue to avoid chemicals and drying heat, nurture your own natural oils, add new ones, use conditioners, and sheen will return.

5. *Split ends.* If your hair has a frizzy halo and instead of lying smoothly looks as if you brushed it in front of a fan, then you've got split ends, a/k/a the "frizzies."

Although the frizzies constitute perhaps *the* most common hair complaint, the medical truth of the matter is that practically nobody was born with them. In almost all cases the frizzies are entirely self-induced by people who are unwittingly damaging the protective cuticles of their own hair, thereby allowing the softer inner structures of the hair in effect to unravel.

I should note here that some people like their frizzies. Afros and supercurly permanents are glorified cases of frizzies that happen to look great. But if your hairstyle doesn't involve an electric halo, then you'll want to do all you can to banish the frizzies.

Your individual hairs moving against one another produce constant friction, which causes electrostatic charges. And hair with ragged cuticles and split ends is *especially* liable to these charges. Because electrically charged hairs repel one another, frizzy heads are defiantly hard to style.

Patients with severe frizzies often complain, "I can't understand it. I do so much for my hair." That over-treatment, of course, is usually the source of the problem. These people should also give their hair a vacation from processes like too-frequent shampooing. Daily washing is okay under normal circumstances, but if your hair is dry and lacks natural oils, or if you aren't giving it needed conditioners, then you can easily *induce* the frizzies. No matter how often you shampoo, the prescription for unfrizzing is to cut down on washings.

One of the biggest causes of split ends is overtreatment with chemical dyes and bleaches. Hair cuticles on various heads will tolerate the peroxide in dyes and bleaches to different degrees, but all chemical treatments will *inevitably* damage the cuticle. A ruined, ragged cuticle not only leads to split ends but also makes hair dull and difficult to manage.

Overmanipulation is another major cause of split ends. Everybody likes nicely styled hair, but overbrushing, over-teasing, too-heavy brushes with *sharp* bristles, or excessive and careless use of brush rollers can all damage the cuticle or even deform the hair. So frequent are these abuses that there are medical names for them. *Pili torti* refers to hair that has been abused, usually by overbrushing. These hairs have normal shafts, but somewhere along each one is a section where the hair is literally jammed into itself. In another condition, called *trichorexis nodosa,* each otherwise normal hair shaft has a little nodule on it. This is just a different response to the abusive brushing or combing that also causes *pili torti.* Then there's *pili spindulosa,* in which the victim has so antagonized his or her hair that each strand has begun to look like a stretched-out spring. A whole headful of hairs suffering from these conditions produces that wild, flyaway look everyone wants to avoid.

Too much heat is another culprit in the war against healthy hair. Electric rollers, curling irons, blow dryers, and hot oil treatments are all okay in moderation, but overuse, *especially of blowers,* can literally scorch the cuticle. Once that cuticle is weakened, the hair shaft is inevitably going to split.

Humidity causes frizzies because of the natural tendency of hair to equilibrate with the water content of the air that surrounds it. If it's a rainy day, your hair is going to suck up water from the air, swell, and make every split end stand out.

If you're fleeing the frizzies, beware of excessive exposure to the sun. The sun's ultraviolet rays can damage the cuticle, and ionizing rays electrostatically charge overdry hairs. Combine blazing sun with a dip in a chlorine-treated pool and/or a swim in a pool followed by a sauna, and the combination of heat dehydration and chlorine attack on the cuticle will frizz even normally healthy hair. Chlorine chemicals are harsh on cuticles and can turn mild frizzies considerably frizzier. Taking a sauna is like sticking your head in an oven. The dry heat further desiccates the hair and leads to flyaway unmanageability.

Artificially dried-out hair isn't solely a result of summer sunshine, swimming, or saunas. During the winter central heating effectively dehumidifies the environment, drying not only skin but hair as well. I observe that very often people with scaly, dry skin eczema also have the frizzies.

The point of all this is not to warn you never again to swim in a chemically chlorinated pool, play golf in the baking sun, occasionally style your hair with a blow dryer, or live in a centrally heated house. But if you have frizzies, these factors will make them worse. We noted earlier that the only real cure for split ends is to cut them off. However, you can improve their appearance and retard the rate of splitting by eliminating abusive practices and properly conditioning the hair as described in Chapter 4.

3

Shampooing

The good news is that the best ways to wash your hair are usually the cheapest. In general there are no bad shampoos, only inappropriate or unduly expensive ones. Shampoos with high price tags usually reflect the cost of big advertising budgets or unnecessary additives like expensive perfume. But do you shampoo to perfume your head or to clean your hair?

American consumers are blessed with an incredibly wide selection of shampoo products. And they take advantage of it: Annual shampoo sales have passed the $200,000,000 mark. The average American shampoos two times a week, but 25 percent of us don't even bother with shampoo, preferring to stick to plain old soap, which is the basic ingredient of most shampoos, anyway. A mild soap, such as **Neutrogena, Ivory, Dove,** or **Caress**, to name only a few, performs for many people just as well as any specific shampoo product.

Soaps, however, are just for cleaning. Shampoos have additional chemical ingredients and are expected not only to clean but also to impart certain cosmetic properties. A shampoo earns points for giving hair luster and manage-ability. It also must be able to clean away natural skin secretions, environmental dirt, the residue of any hair products, dandruff, and skin debris without leaving the hair so clean that it's unmanageable. Fortunately most shampoos do this quite well. After a normal shampoo you can expect anywhere from 65 percent to 90 percent of the total extractable oil on your hair still to be there. If it weren't, your hair would look wildly dry and flyaway.

These days, shampoos come in liquid, cream, lotion, gel, aerosol, and powder forms. The last two are usually made out of talcum powder, whereas all the others have essentially the same basic ingredient—soap. If a shampoo manufacturer no longer bases his formula on soap, it's only because he's substituted an even cheaper chemical-detergent base.

Whether your hair is dry or normal or oily no longer poses any particular shampoo problem, since most products are available in different forms for each type of hair. The varying formulas usually boil down to adding a little oil or lanolin to the dry-hair product and extracting a little from the oily one.

You must experiment with various shampoos, since there is simply no alternative to trial and error if you want to find the ideal product for your hair. The purpose of this chapter is to explain potential shampoo shortcomings by placing them in the demythologized context of hard medical facts instead of silly commercial claims.

WHAT'S IN A SHAMPOO?

Remember that no shampoo is going to make your hair fall out even if you use it every day. From a cosmetic standpoint, shampooing daily is actually a good idea, unless you're suffering from extreme dryness or split ends. Of course, the main ingredient of every shampoo, except spray powders, is either soap or some type of chemical detergent. So-called organic formulas are just as soapy as their less pretentious sisters.

In addition to a soap base, the average shampoo contains a host of multisyllabic chemical additives, included for various purposes. *Foam builders* are among the most commonly used since the media have successfully convinced the consuming public that you can't clean anything without lots of suds. Actually, many substances clean effectively without much foaming, but it's still comforting to have a headful of rich lather, hence foam builders. Not only do they ensure lots of thick lather, they also make the shampoo easy to rinse out of your hair.

Sequestering agents are chemicals that attract calcium, lime, and other minerals. They make water "hard," and hard water hampers good lather. So, in the same way people install water softeners, many manufacturers put sequestering agents into their shampoo formulas to trap these minerals. Hard water isn't a universal problem, but where it is, these softening agents do indeed make both sudsing and rinsing considerably easier.

Paramount among shampoo additives is *conditioner*. Conditioners combat unwanted fluffiness and lubricate the hair shaft, but a conditioner that's great on one person's hair may make another's oily or lusterless. Again, the universal prescription is trial and error.

Many popular shampoos also contain either *opacifying* or *clarifying agents*. When a manufacturer doesn't think a product looks "sexy" enough in its naturally transparent state, a chemical agent is added to cloud it. Similarly, clarifying agents transform cloudy formulas into clear substances. It is important to note that neither opacifiers nor clarifiers affect the cleaning or conditioning of your hair.

Since many shampoo ingredients encourage the growth of molds and bacteria, the last major ingredient is *preservative*.

Again, preservatives do nothing for your hair, but they do protect what is in the bottle, most importantly, the conditioner.

WHAT IS pH?

Despite all the ballyhoo, the importance of pH balance in shampoo is almost negligible, a clear-cut case of marketing experts cashing in on the heightened ecological consciousness of the public.

Many chemical substances can be described as either acidic or alkaline. For example, orange juice is acidic, but vinegar is more acidic; soap is alkaline, but oven cleaner is more alkaline.

A clinical measure of *acidity* or *alkalinity*, pH is calibrated on a scale of 1 to 14. For example, a pH of 1 means that a substance is extremely acid; pH 7 is neutral, or balanced; and pH 14 is completely alkaline. Orange juice has a low pH; normal skin and hair have a pH of 4.5 to 5.5; water is pH 7; lye or oven cleaner is pH 14.

Advertising copywriters have been flogging pH for all it's worth in recent years, but their claims are only half-truths. To understand fully how the pH factor relates to shampooing and conditioning, one must understand its effect on the hair's imbrications. A hair cuticle is composed of countless tiny scales, called imbrications, which overlap like house shingles, hinged to open or close. Alkaline substances, such as soap and shampoo, will cause the imbrications to open, and when imbrications unhinge, hair becomes hard to manage and dull, since the cortex is then vulnerable to damage. In contrast, acidic substances such as conditioners and cream rinses shut imbrications and make hair shinier by keeping the cortex safely protected.

If this were the whole story, it would make a compelling case for protecting one's hair with "pH-balanced"—acidic or

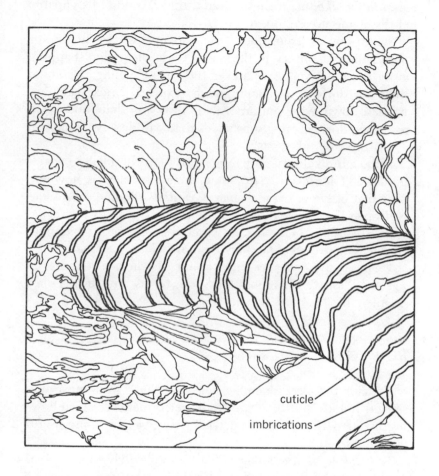

2) A microscopically enlarged strand of hair, highlighting the cuticles and imbrications.

"nonalkaline"—shampoos. However, most shampoos, including the so-called nonalkaline varieties, are soap- and/or detergent-based. Since most soaps and detergents are essentially alkaline; it therefore follows that *most shampoos are*

essentially alkaline; if they weren't, they wouldn't be capable
of dissolving grease, oil, or dirt.

Since this is true, the very concept of an acidic or
nonalkaline shampoo is illogical. Acids clean by stripping
away the top layer of whatever they are cleaning: Diamond
rings are dipped in cleaning acids; exposed brick walls are
washed down with muriatic acid. But your hair and scalp
tissue requires cleaning substances that will dissolve, not strip
away, dirt and oil.

Although alkalinity is detergent by nature, alkaline shampoos won't hurt your hair, since their harshness is nowhere
near that of lye or oven cleaner. Granted, alkaline substances
will open the imbrications, but that effect is easily corrected
with a conditioner or cream rinse. Remember, if shampoos
weren't slightly alkaline, they couldn't clean your hair.

I would advise you to forget about pH during your search
for the "ideal" shampoo—all such terms are finally just
double-talk.

HOW TO BUY A SHAMPOO

To find the best shampoo for your hair, you must buy
several brands and compare their performance. The following list of performance properties will give you some useful
guidelines.

1. *Quality of the lather.* There is no single standard of
quality, since billowy lather is *not* necessarily synonymous
with good cleaning. If your locality has very hard water, a
shampoo with a good sequestering agent will ensure plenty
of suds. If you don't get enough lather, either the shampoo
does not have a sequestering agent or it has a poor one. Since
sequestering agents are not listed on shampoo labels, you'll
have to experiment with different products if lather is
important.

2. *Detergency.* The most desirable level of detergency, or alkaline cleaning strength, depends on your hair type and its level of oiliness. The shampoo you ultimately choose should clean your hair without making it unduly dry. By the way, shampooing will not affect permanent hair dyes.

3. *Rinsability.* You should expect a good shampoo to rinse out in less than a minute, or two if your hair is very long.

4. *Conditioning action.* A good shampoo will leave the hair soft, shining, easy to comb, and able to hold a style.

5. *Lubricity.* A shampoo's ability to prevent tangles and to make the individual hairs slip by one another easily is known as lubricity, which is determined by the unique combination of your hair and any given shampoo. Maximizing the effect is purely a matter of personal experimentation.

6. *Body building.* Shampoos that add body do so by coating the individual hairs with variations of protein, which makes thin, fine hair look thicker. You can, however, get more effective body-building results by using a separate protein conditioner after you shampoo (see Chapter 4).

Unless you're just mad about the smell or dazzled by a certain designer label, I urge you not to spend extra money on expensive scented shampoos. The same advice applies to esoteric formulas, special "organic" preparations, and products that make grand pH claims.

The following recommended shampoos all do a good job and are mostly quite reasonably priced. **Breck** and **Prell** are hard to beat for lots of lather and reasonable price. Breck (all varieties) is additionally good for tinted or colored hair. I like **Conti** not only because of the reasonable price but because it contains lanolin and olive oil, both very good for dry hair. **Revlon Milk Plus 6** contains an old standby protein conditioner, milk, which makes it good for hair that needs body. I like **Earthborn** not for all its pH claims but because it smells so good. **Pantene**, made by the same company that makes the tranquilizer Valium, is not cheap, but it contains pantothenic acid, a good protein conditioner and body builder. **Alberto VO5** is a part of American culture by now, and it's very good for dry hair. **Johnson Baby Shampoo** is mild and appeals to everyone, from models to football players, as does Clairol's protein-enriched **Great Body**.

For particularly greasy or oily hair, you might try **Fitch** or **Toni's Lemon-Up**. They'll both leave hair squeaky clean, and Toni's product has a very pleasing lemon scent. If you're a highly allergic type, liable to sudden red bumps and rashes, Johnson & Johnson makes a product called **Purpose**, which is expensive but superhypoallergenic. If you have dull and/or gray hair, you might try **Bright Side**, which is neither a bleach nor a dye but adds highlights to dull hair via a galaxy of chemical ingredients.

When there's no time to shampoo but you have to, anyway, try one of the dry shampoos, **Minipoo** or **Pssssst**. This sort of product is a temporary measure only, and cannot be used as a regular shampoo. It doesn't do any cleaning at all, but since it is based on oil-absorbing powder, it will improve the appearance of hair that's very oily—at least until there's time to shampoo properly.

Finally, many big drug chains and discount houses bottle their own inexpensive shampoos. They're bargains and highly recommended. And don't forget plain **Palmolive** and other bathroom soaps—**Dial, Dove, Ivory, Woodbury**. They work very well for many people, so well, in fact, that there is even a product on the market called **Soap Shampoo**.

HOW TO SHAMPOO

No matter *what* the label says, lather only once. Unless your hair is literally dripping with natural oil, two latherings will strip away too much of it. This will result in unmanageability, from wide-open imbrications, and/or excessive dryness, from too much oil depletion.

If you want to, it is perfectly safe to shampoo normal and oily hair every day. Hair won't fall out from too much shampooing. Hard water can turn shampooing into a problem by making the hair hard to lather and harder to rinse. Water softeners help; so do shampoos with sequestering agents; in extreme cases you might want to use soft spring bottled water from the supermarket. No matter what water you use, make sure it's hot—not scalding, not cool, just plain old hot.

If you have naturally attractive hair and don't care to pay for fancy packaging or corporate advertising budgets, go ahead and wash your hair with soap. If your hair is dry but you love your soap or shampoo anyway, try adding a teaspoon of olive oil to the lather. If that makes your hair too oily, use less; if your hair's still too dry, try a bit more; do not put olive or any other oil into your shampoo bottle in advance, since the product probably won't have the necessary preservatives to avoid spoilage.

Just as you can add a simple household item like olive oil for dryness, so you can add household proteins for body. Again, don't add them to the bottle, because of the spoilage problem. To add body to thin and/or fine hair, take a cup of milk with you into the shower, combine it with the shampoo lather, give it a minute to sink in, then rinse. You can also try egg whites or unflavored gelatine, both of which are protein substances that will coat the hair shafts and make your hair look fuller.

Aside from additives for dryness and body, there are no special shampoo instructions for the other types of hair. In every case thorough rinsing is necessary to flush out completely the lather, dirt, and excess oil. Shampoos are primarily just for cleaning; they condition the hair to make it more manageable but only to a limited degree. Advice for people whose hair needs substantially more body or protection is contained in the next chapter.

4

Conditioning

All conditioners and cream-rinse products are essentially mildly acidic, just as all shampoos are essentially alkaline, so the concept of nonalkalinity *is* meaningful after you've finished your shampoo. If your shampooed hair looks dull because of imbrications opened by shampoo alkalinity, then an acid conditioner will close these imbrications and both restore and enhance the hair's natural sheen. Incidentally, the terms "conditioner" and "cream-rinse" refer to approximately the same type of preparation. "Cream rinse" simply means a type of conditioner that's applied to the hair in a liquid form.

The effect of an acid-pH conditioner on the cuticle is to close the imbrications. This not only protects the inner hair structure but also imparts shine and luster to the hair's surface. Good salons usually follow a shampoo with a simple acid conditioning rinse. You can make an equally effective acid rinse at home with the following formula: Take three tablespoons of either apple-cider vinegar or lemon juice, mix into a glass of cool water, comb the mixture through freshly shampooed wet hair, and rinse with cool water. This makes hair shine.

In addition to closing the imbrications with an acid pH, nearly all conditioners contain some form of protein. Protein coats the hair shaft, gives it body, and makes it easy to manage with brush and comb. Balsam, an aromatic oily substance derived from the tree of the same name, milk, soy, egg whites, gelatin, an exotic vegetable called a tong bean, and the placenta of cattle and sheep are all common examples of protein well suited to the hair. Because of their coating action, protein conditioners are particularly important to fine and/or limp hair that lacks fullness. But they're also a great help to thick, dry hair that tends to be electric and unbrushable after a shampoo.

Conditioners were developed to help particularly bad problems of dullness, split ends, flyaway hair, lack of body, and postshampoo tangles. Since many shampoo products— especially in recent years—have added conditioning agents that adequately deal with these problems, the separate step of conditioning may sometimes be like gilding the lily. For example, your shampoo may raise your imbrications so minimally as to leave your hair perfectly beautiful and lustrous and with no need for an acid rinse. Or it may already contain protein, which gives enough body to slightly fine or thin hair and makes a protein cream rinse superfluous. Or your shampoo may contain an oil, such as lanolin, that imparts all the manageability your hair needs without making any antitangle cream rinse necessary.

The point here—as regards protein—is that often there is either no reason to put any on or to do so would be superfluous. It's a matter of personal experimentation.

It's easy enough to add protein to hair at home simply by adding a cup of milk or the whites of two eggs to your shampoo lather. But this protein differs from that in commercially prepared shampoos and conditioners because it is not what is called "substantive protein." In order to be substantive, the protein must be processed into smaller molecules, which supposedly can better penetrate the hair. An American Medical Association's 1976 publication called "Skin and Hair Care" quaintly describes trying to condition the hair with nonsubstantive proteins as being like forcing a bowling ball into a grape. This is funny, but it is not the gospel truth.

The longer the hairstyle, the greater chance of split ends. The ends of short hair are younger; the cuticles have had less exposure and are consequently in better condition. Long-hair ends are older, and the cuticles have inevitably sustained more wear and tear. The popular resurgence of long hair and the introduction of high-powered electric blow dryers have combined to bring on an epidemic of split ends. If you're one of the victims, your salvation is an effective protein conditioner. But even if you have normal, healthy hair, conditioners will make it shinier.

Beer is a carbohydrate and contains little protein. I know of little in beer that can give body to hair, and it is also doubtful whether or not it improves manageability. It does make your hair smell like an old can of beer, which is why I think it is a superlatively bad thing to put on your head.

BUYING A CONDITIONER

The three major functions of conditioners are as follows:

1. To coat the individual hairs with protein, thereby adding body and sealing in moisture;

2. To separate the hairs from one another, prevent buildup of electrostatic charge, and make the hairs easy to comb or brush; and

3. To close the imbrications opened by shampoos, bleaches, and other chemicals, thereby smoothing the cuticle surface and inducing sheen.

Determining how often to condition is purely a matter of personal experimentation. Although you can't cause any harm by overconditioning, too much coating can make hair look and feel oily, which defeats the purpose of adding fullness. Some people keep a bottle of conditioner in the shower and follow daily shampoos with brief conditioning treatments consisting of a minute on the head and a minute of rinsing. Other people condition once a week with one of the home packs described on the pages that follow. Personal regimens are a matter of individual convenience and hair condition. Regardless of *how* you do your conditioning, you'll be doing it for the purposes listed above. And if you *don't* need help along those lines, don't bother with conditioners. Many people, after all, do go through life doing nothing to or for their hair except washing it, and they look just fine.

It is not my intention here to list every product on the market. The following conditioners are good, and they're representative of what's available. For convenience, I've included a short description of how each is used.

We'll start with **Maintain**, the Cadillac of conditioners. It calls itself the revitalizing lotion and is applied to towel-dried shampooed hair; no need to rinse it out, just let it dry on the head. Maintain is used at least twice a week or whenever you shampoo. It's not cheap; if Coke cost this much, you'd pay thirty dollars per bottle.

Elizabeth Arden's Especially Effective Hair Conditioner describes itself as a creamy reconditioner. It's excellent for problems of static, tangles, and dullness. Again, it's applied to towel-dried shampooed hair. You finger-comb it in, then rinse with lukewarm water.

Phinal Phase, by Redkin, is a very reasonably priced acid-balance cream rinse, great for adding shine and manageability. You mix it with water, shake well, then rub the mixture in with your fingers and don't rinse out.

L'Oréal's Oleocap was formulated for overbleached or overblown hair that suffers from dullness and bad frizzies. It's a kit, complete with applicator bottle. You immerse the bottle in hot water, then work the heated contents into a lather on unshampooed hair. After that you wrap your hair, lather and all, in a damp hot towel for ten minutes, then shampoo as usual. L'Oréal advises that you use this conditioner after every swim in a chlorinated pool and before every shampoo.

Clairol makes several excellent and reasonably priced conditioners. The first is **Conditioner Beauty Pack**, whose contents are supposed to be left on the hair for twenty to thirty minutes before rinsing. I think that the hair just can't absorb anything more after ten minutes, but leave it on if you want. This product is designed for general reconditioning, which means it's good for dullness, damage, split ends and limpness.

Clairol also makes **Long and Silky**, "for girls who never want to cut their hair." The big advantage of Long and Silky is that it can be applied for sixty seconds, then rinsed out immediately.

Also by Clairol is a product called **Buttermilk**. This is an organic formula with an acid pH of 6. It's applied to clean, towel-dried hair and rinsed out after a few minutes. The acid pH really makes a difference here. In the absence of alkaline soaps for cleaning, it closes the imbrications and enhances the hair's appearance.

Alberto VO5 makes a hot oil treatment that involves heating tubes of the product in hot water, then massaging the contents into hot wet hair until it lathers. This is followed first by a rinse, then by your regular shampoo.

Borghese Herbal Blend Conditioning Hair Pack contains chamomile, fennel, and sage. It's good for sheen and manageability and is applied to the hair after shampooing.

Next is a product that advertises a "secret Danish formula." It's called **Unicure**, has a nice acid pH that locks the cuticles shut, and claims to be good even for the skin.

Helena Rubinstein makes an ingenious product called **Hair**

Care Problem Solver. It's a shampoo, but it contains soluble beads of conditioner that float undissolved in the liquid until they interact with water on your head. Rubinstein also makes a product called **Skin Dew**, which is applied to hair after the shampoo and is not rinsed out.

Palm Beach Firm and Fill contains animal placenta. This one requires wrapping your lathered head in a hot towel and sitting for a bit. But there's no doubt that it effectively coats and conditions frizzy hair.

Also good is **Vidal Sassoon's Protein Cream Hair Remoisturizer.** This is applied after the shampoo, then rinsed out. Sassoon also has a protein pack treatment in which the hair is wrapped with a hot towel before rinsing.

Finally, I want to mention **Braggi Hair and Scalp Conditioner.** Although this is promoted primarily for men, it is an excellent postshampoo conditioner for both sexes. Again, it's one of those which are not rinsed out.

Please note that almost any commercially prepared conditioner or cream rinse with protein, an acid pH, and/or oils of any sort will condition your hair. This includes cheap discount chain-store house brands. Although you can't actually overcondition hair, saturation with protein will make it difficult to bleach, dye, and sometimes even to shampoo.

No conditioner or cream rinse can do magic with one application. You must make conditioning a regular practice. The underlying concept is to protect those hair cuticles. Once you've mastered that, you'll assure yourself of shining, full-bodied hair.

5

Blow Dryers

There is a decided difference between styling hair in an attractive shape and simply blowing it dry after a shampoo. Good styling requires a good haircut. However, with hot-air blow dryers, the very act of drying gives the hair a fullness which in itself is an act of styling.

Because hair is malleable when exposed to heat, blow dryers make it easy to remove unwanted curls and waves and/or to add them where they're wanted. So appliances that started out as simple hair dryers have also become home styling tools complete with special nozzles to direct the air stream, brushes to pull out natural curls, and other features.

Because of the nature of hair, drying and styling are a natural combination. Keratin, the substance which consti-tutes hair, is essentially pure protein. And like all proteins, hair can be heat-treated to change its shape. By way of illustration, consider a rod of steel. Steel isn't a protein, of course, but when it's heated, it can be bent or molded. Protein gelatin is also malleable when heated, and it also maintains its molded shape when cool. It is the like capacity of protein-structured hair, namely, to change shape when heated, that has stimulated the wide use of blow dryers for purposes other than just drying.

The problem with all appliances that blow hot air onto hair is that they are extremely drying. Used too often, they can make hair dull, brittle, and filled with split ends. Fifteen minutes of scorching hot air blasts after every shower will inevitably cause progressive, cumulative damage, first to the cuticle, then to the inner hair structure. Hair which has been regularly blown dry for a prolonged period of time becomes progressively more wretched: The unnaturally high heat of blow drying not only makes individual hairs look dry but can also burn the scalp and even kill hair follicles.

The problem with hair-blower abuse is twofold. First there's the hard-to-resist lure of easily obtained fullness. This is complicated by a second factor, the American urge to buy the "bigger and better" model. When it comes to hair dryers, small is definitely better. Overwatted blowers, namely, those with more than 1,000 watts, should be avoided. Of course, the more powerful the appliance, the faster it dries your hair. But take my advice: Go slow, be patient. Fast drying is simply not worth the risk of damaging the hair.

I would advise against daily use of any blow dryer. If you have a hairstyle that must be blown out to look good, then for the sake of long-term health and appearance of your hair, I would strongly urge you to change your style. I know how many people depend on blow dryers—and I know this is a bit like crying out in the wilderness—but the fact remains that blow drying is bad for hair. If you use a blow dryer only occasionally, that's one thing. But I would not get into the habit of using it either to dry hair after shampooing or to prepare your regular daily hairstyle.

If you do decide to get a dryer for occasional styling, there are all sorts of things to consider prior to purchase. All blow dryers work on the same basic principle: A small fan blows air over a heated electrical coil. Most of them also have at least two speed settings, two heat settings, and various coarse and fine brush and comb attachments. But there the similarities end.

Assuming you have directed your search to products with hair-saving wattage under 1,000 (this information is clearly marked on the appliance itself), you should next look for the Underwriters Laboratories' seal. This organization tests the safety of all cord electric appliances, and I don't think you should buy any electrical product that doesn't bear its seal of approval. UL also assures that there is a thermostat to shut the appliance off if the nozzle temperature exceeds 150° F.

Next, check that there is a screen on the air-intake port. Hair has a habit of being sucked against the port during drying, and unless there's a screen it can become painfully and exasperatingly tangled in the fan. Fortunately, most models now make this standard equipment.

Before you buy any blower or styler, take it out of the box and turn it on. Some of these gadgets are unbelievably noisy. Some are uncomfortably heavy, have handles that are difficult to grasp, or vibrate so much they cause your whole arm to tingle unpleasantly. Usually the cords are short, but some are ridiculously so. You should not only look for at least a ten-foot cord but also try to find a model whose cord is detachable for easy storage. Other useful features include travel bags, attached hooks or rings that let you hang the appliance on the wall, and built-in water misters to facilitate styling.

Since a blow dryer vibrates so much, you should never set it down while it's running. The vibrations can make the appliance creep right off the edge of whatever you set it on. And very few blowers will survive a fall from waist height without substantial and usually disabling damage. If you drop any small electrical appliance, for safety's sake it's best to have it examined as soon as possible even if it still seems to work okay.

Following is a list of reasonably priced, solidly built blow dryers with most—if not all—of the features recommended above. As with any list, there's always going to be a new product coming out and an old one discontinued. How long does a hair blower last? If you use the average blower fifteen minutes a day (and by all means, don't!), it has a statistical life span of one year. Here are some good ones:

> Clairol AB-1
> Clairol AB-2
> General Electric SD-1
> General Electric SD-2
> General Electric STC1
> GE Zoom 'n Groom D1-PD-1
> Gillette THD-2
> Gillette THD-2A
> Hamilton Beach 423
> Lady Schick 338
> Lady Schick Speed Styler 352
> Norelco Shape 'n Dry 750 HB6600
> Northern 1800
> Panasonic EH-741
> Panasonic EH-745
> Remington HW-3
> Remington HW-6
> Remington 600 PD600
> Schick 336
> Sunbeam EC-5
> Sunbeam EC-6

RANDOM THOUGHTS ON HAIR DRYING

Hand-held blow dryers and beauty-parlor hoods both employ the principle of rapid evaporation. But the hand-held blowers are considerably hotter than the hood dryers in beauty parlors because they don't cover the whole head.

Irreversible damage can occur whenever hair is subjected to heat in excess of 150° F. This damage can include scorching, brittleness, unmanageability, and loss of shine. More hair damage stems, however, from overmanipulation while drying than from excessive heat. Fancy flips or aggressive teasing under a blower can effect a dramatic style, all right, but it will weaken the hair.

DR. ZIZMOR'S CHECKLIST FOR PEOPLE WHO USE BLOW DRYERS

1. Don't use your blower for daily drying: save it for occasional styling. Once a week won't hurt you. And when you *do* use it, towel dry the wet hair, and comb it before you begin styling.

2. Avoid a hairstyle that requires daily blow drying to look good. Beware of any dependence on blowers to make hair look full.

3. If you're going to buy a dryer, get one with low wattage (under 1,000). Or use the low heat setting on the higher-watt models.

4. Protect your hair while blow drying with one of the heat-activated blow-dry conditioners. Protein-based products are now available specifically for the purpose of coating the hair and protecting it from the intense heat of a blower. Clairol makes a liquid product called **Zap**, as well as a spray called **Kindness**. Pantene manufactures a good liquid called **The Heat Solution**. And Cosmetco makes another called **Blow-Care**. Each of these products requires only a single combed-through application after shampooing and requires no rinsing out.

5. Start using the blower first at the *back* of the head. Do the roots first, then the middle. Always save curling and styling the ends for last.

6

Home Styling and Grooming

Nobody can teach you how to style your own hair. Styling is an artistic talent and is almost always left to professional haircutters (see Chapter 11). What *you* can do is keep your hair in good condition and enhance a good cut with the following appliances and cosmetic preparations.

HAIR APPLIANCES

As for blow dryers, we've already measured their ability to train the hair and make it look full-bodied against the drying dangers they pose when used regularly. But used no more than once a week, they shouldn't cause any noticeable damage in either the short or the long run.

Recently other appliances have become almost as popular as blow dryers. A good example is the renascent curling iron. By the late 1930s, most curling irons were gathering dust in attics. But about a dozen years ago, they were tentatively reintroduced and today are again widely available. Curling irons are used only on dry hair, and they're great for adding a flip or touching up a wilted hairdo. The modern models are thermostatically controlled to ensure correct heat automatically and protect against the burns that plagued the curly-coiffed beauties of yesteryear. What's more, today's curling irons have special coatings to prevent hair from sticking to the iron, sometimes even push-button misters.

As with anything else, you can overuse a curling iron. But when employed moderately for occasional dressy curls, it can't hurt you. Features to look for include a swivel base on the electric cord; a long cord; an Underwriters Laboratories seal, and a well-designed stand that allows you to put the iron down and pick it up easily while it's hot. Of the irons I've seen, I like **Crazy Curl** by Clairol (Model 200), **Lady Shick Quick Curls** (Model C1-1), and the **Oster Mist Set** (Model 381-OSAB).

You won't catch the Cosmo girl letting "him" see her set her hair in curlers anymore. In fact, almost no one sleeps with curlers, at least not since electric rollers were invented. Both General Electric and Clairol make electric hair-setting kits that combine heat and moisture to set hair. Let me emphasize that setting is not the same as styling. For any set to look its best, it must be done on a well-cut head of hair. Electric rollers themselves aren't electrified; rather, they are heated and moisturized in a carrier box, then transferred individually to your hair. To be sure, there's a technique to be learned, but they're fast and they work just as well as a whole night in the old nonelectric models. Be sure to let the hair cool completely before brushing, otherwise you'll weaken the set.

A very popular appliance for people with curly or kinky hair is the hot comb, which will be discussed in detail in Chapter 7. For now I'll note that hot combs are used in conjunction with hot oils only for straightening. They work well, at least temporarily. But there is a danger of damaging the hair follicles if too much hot oil gets onto the scalp.

Many people with curly hair straighten it by the time-honored method of ironing. The household iron is hardly a new beauty appliance, but I want to say that with proper caution and moderate skill, hair can be ironed straight with good results. If you're careful and keep the iron at the low end of the "warm" setting, it may not pose any more of a threat to your hair than a blow dryer; however, I do not recommend it.

HAIR-GROOMING PREPARATIONS

Since hair falls into various categories, a hair dressing can be good without necessarily being good for everybody. Hair dressings all aspire to the same general goals: to make hair easier to manage, to impart sheen and luster without greasiness, and to provide some degree of protection from the rain, wind, and other elements. To get the best results, you must use a product that's designed for your type of hair, which is where most people become confused.

The majority of hair-grooming-product customers have dry, dull, hard-to-manage hair. Every hair follicle has its own oil gland to provide natural grooming oils and to prevent this situation, but as I've mentioned, the natural oil flow is easily interrupted by excessive bleaching, dyeing, overwashing, etc. Under these conditions the hair needs supplemental oil. Any type of oil will do—animal, vegetable, or mineral.

The addition of oil won't help brittleness, but it will make dry hair more lustrous and manageable. You can also further enhance the moisturizing properties of the oil-based grooming products listed below by wetting the hair before applying them. The oil in the dressing will tend to seal in the moisture on each hair shaft after your hair is dry.

Traditional merchandising techniques have tended to restrict hair-care products to one sex or the other. If ever there was a truly unisex family of products, it's those for hair care. I want to stress here that women should feel completely free to use certain hair dressings even if they're packaged and promoted for men. Witness the recent public acceptance of hair sprays for men. Not very long ago, a man who used a hair spray could count on being the butt of insulting jokes, but no longer. Now it's time for women to realize that their hair may well respond beautifully to male-associated things like brilliantine or pomade. These very oily products are especially good for the many women who overwash or overprocess their hair.

If your hair is thick but dull and dry, I highly recommend **Alberto VO5**. This product—the best seller in the United States—adds highlights and control. It comes in varying strengths, all of them very oily. You can also use VO5—or, for that matter, any other oily dressing—in lieu of a conditioner. Squeeze about an inch from the tube, work it into the hair, leave it on for a half hour, and then shampoo. The final rinse leaves enough VO5 in the hair to ensure manageability.

Clairol's Vitapointe is another good dressing for thick, dull, dry, flyaway hair. It's made from a formula based on mineral oil and beeswax and is a bit less greasy than VO5. Also very effective are **Wildroot** and **Brylcreem**. Usually a *very* small dab of any of these products, spread on the palm and worked into the hair, will be enough. You'll have to experiment to determine how much of a dab your own hair requires.

You can also make your own hair dressing by working less than a teaspoon of olive oil or any other type of household oil into your hair. Some people take olive oil, add a few drops of perfume, and use the solution as a dip for a comb. Alternatively, products associated with skin care can be just as effective on dry hair. A little dab of **Vaseline** or **Aqua-phore** can make your dry hair just as lustrous as a dab of Brylcreem.

Whatever you use, beware of buildup. Overly dry hair is an invitation to excessive use of oily hair dressings, but making formerly dry hair too oily is no improvement. Besides, when the hair is too oily, there's always a risk of *pomade acne*, pimple flare-ups at the hairline caused by too much pore-clogging oil. This danger is particularly acute for younger people and slowly tapers off after age thirty.

Almost everybody can use a little grooming. In our alternately air-conditioned and centrally heated world even normal and slightly oily hair can become dry.

There are various greaseless gels on the market for hair that is not terribly dry but in need of some grooming. My favorite is called **Drest**. This product looks and smells great, contains an antidandruff agent, and is reactivated every time you run a wet comb through your hair. Also good is **Groom 'n Clean**, another greaseless gel. Or perhaps you might want to experiment with **Score**, a greaseless product whose alcohol base is good for people who don't need oil supplements. Score, along with tonics like **Vitalis** and **Pinot,** are two of the products firmly established in most minds as being strictly for men. However, this is simply a misconception. They make combing and brushing easier, impart an attractive sheen, and are highly recommended for all normal to slightly oily hair that's being dulled by environmental factors.

If your hair is very oily, you don't need any hair dressing. Problem oiliness is best dealt with by means of an effective shampoo. Likewise, limp or thin hair doesn't need a grooming product as much as it needs the protein body builders contained in conditioners and certain shampoos. You might also try **Pantene** or **Thickit**, two products containing protein that will give a full-bodied look to thinning hair between shampoos.

If your hairstyle is the least bit complicated, then you are probably already using a hair spray. At this writing, ecological pressures seem at last to be winning the battle against ozone-depleting spray-can propellants. This means that there will undoubtedly be many changes in the products listed below. At the same time, the need for fine-spray lacquer plasticizers is not likely to fade. And some manufacturers already have new "ecological" holding sprays in fine-mist pumps on the drugstore shelves.

In my opinion hair sprays are very similar to one another. For that reason I'd stick to the cheaper sprays, since additional price doesn't bring much additional quality. I'd also recommend that you use "regular hold" whether or not your hair seems to need "strong hold." The strong sprays have too many strong, drying chemicals that can potentially damage your hair cuticles. If you need extra holding power, it's better to use more "regular." Of course, if your style holds with just a hair dressing, then by all means skip the spray.

Hair sprays are divided into two categories: plain sprays and conditioning sprays. Among the many plain sprays available, I like **Breck, Clairol Final Net, Gillette's Dry Look, Alberto VO5, Self-Styling Adorn**, and **L'Oréal's Elnett**, to name only a representative few. Conditioning sprays contain oils or proteins, but I seriously doubt that much conditioner can be effectively applied to the hair with a spray. Nonetheless, it's still possible your hair might respond particularly well to any one of the sprays in this category. For example, I like **Protein 29, Allercreme** (which is hypo-allergenic and might really be valuable, given the many people who have allergic reactions to their hair sprays), **Marcelle** (also hypoallergenic), **Redkin,** and **Hairspray de Pantene** (which contains a "secret Swiss" agent, probably the protein called pantothenic acid).

COMBING AND BRUSHING

We come now to the technical-sounding subject of *traction alopecia,* a widely observed condition of temporary hair loss caused by tugging! Traction alopecia is amazingly common, although I doubt that more than 3 percent of the public has ever heard of it. Put simply, it means yanking out your own hair. You can suffer from traction alopecia as a result of excessive combing and brushing, overly tight rubber bands, kerchiefs, rollers, and any practice or hairstyle that causes the hair to be pulled back tightly for prolonged periods of time.

Hair loss from traction alopecia usually occurs on the sides of the head. The proper diagnosis is also typically rejected as absurd by many patients. But if you are experiencing noticeable hair loss on the temples or above the ears, you should immediately discontinue any hairstyle that involves pulling the hair severely back. Braids and barrettes can do as much damage as rubber bands. Using them occasionally certainly can't hurt you. But prolonged use *can* very often pull the hair right out. Fortunately the loss is usually temporary, and when the cause is eliminated, the hair will quickly grow back.

As I've pointed out, traction alopecia can also be the result of too much brushing. The tradition of brushing for 100 strokes a day is not good for your hair. I'd make 25 strokes the absolute limit.

Hair loss from brushing happens, but it is not a matter of bristle type. Many people extol the virtue of pure natural bristle over the cheaper nylon varieties. The real culprits are brushes that are too heavy, brushers whose strokes are too forceful, and bristles with ends that are *too sharp*. Sharp bristles fracture hair and damage hair cuticles. Make sure your bristle ends are *rounded* and blunt and it won't matter what variety of bristle you use. I see no inherent advantage to expensive pure bristle over cheaper nylon. Before you buy any brush, comb, or plastic styling brush, test it against your palm. If the bristles are sharp and spiky, don't buy that brush.

The real point of brushing the hair is to distribute natural scalp oils along the length of each hair. The best way to do this is to let the head hang between the knees and brush from the back of the neck forward. Also important is to brush all the way to the end of the hair, so that the natural grooming oils are fully distributed.

It's a bad idea to brush from front to back in front of a mirror because of the ease with which one can drop into a light trance and overbrush. Brushing is a natural outlet for aggression. The larger the brush, the more aggression gets taken out on the hair, and that can lead to traction alopecia.

What applies to brushes also applies to combs. I would advise everybody to use the widest-toothed comb available, for the simple reason that wide teeth pull out fewer hairs. Any comb is fine; there's no medical reason to prefer one over another, just as long as the teeth are widely spaced and the tips are blunt. Neither brushing nor combing will increase circulation on the scalp or do anything else to improve hair growth. But, as with brushing, remember to comb with moderation.

7

Hair Care for Black People

Bushy, springy hair theoretically evolved as a response to equatorial living conditions. Compared to Caucasian hair, it provides better sun protection while maximizing ventilation. But what once was ideally suited has long ago become diluted through migration and intermarriage. Many black people have straight and/or untypically colored hair, and many white people have extremely curly and bushy hair. This is because the world gene pool has become so mixed.

Although hair genes overlap to an extent between races, certain unique structural distinctions do exist. If you were to magnify typical black, Caucasian, and Oriental hairs in cross section, each would have a different shape. The cross section of the Caucasian hair would look almost like a circle. The cross section of the black hair would look like a crescent moon. The Oriental-hair cross section would have a kidney shape.

The flatter the shaft of hair, the curlier the wave pattern. Black people usually have hair so flat and with such a strong wave pattern that it begins curling as soon as it leaves the follicle. Black hair shafts also contain many more air bubbles than those of Caucasians or Orientals. These air bubbles diffuse and refract light, giving the hair a natural matte look instead of a glossy shine. The combination of natural curl and matte look is what accounts for the extreme popularity of oily pomade hair dressings that lubricate the shaft, impart sheen, and make the hair manageable.

What black hair needs most is lots of regular washing, combing, and brushing to avoid growth into the scalp. Besides ingrown hair, the most common hair complaint among black people is scalp dryness and/or lack of shine. Whether your dryness stems from the strong chemicals used in straightening or from the natural matte appearance of the hair, the solution is to add oil.

Almost any oily hair groomer will have excellent results on dull-looking black hair. There are no special hair products just for black people. This is true even though many products are marketed as if they were only for blacks. In practice, anything that adds oil to the hair will give it sheen and manageability. These products are all greasy to touch, but you don't have to use much. And they don't cause an unpleasant greasy appearance. **Vitapointe** is a good popular grooming oil. Pomades like **Dixie Peach, Ultra Sheen Conditioner and Hair Dress, Dax, Duke, Afro Sheen Hair Spray** (which is an oil conditioner and not a holding spray), and, for that matter, plain old **Vaseline** all are excellent. For shampoos, conditioners, and holding hair sprays, use the same products already recommended elsewhere in this book.

The natural spiraling of black hair gives it lots of inherent strength as well as the ability to hold all sorts of styles.

The first black American hairdresser was Madame C. J. Walker, a self-made millionairess, proprietress of a palatial mansion on the Hudson River, and the inventor of the hot comb. Madame Walker was literally a pioneer in the field of modern black beauty care, and her hot combs are used today in much the same way they were when she introduced them, about the turn of the century.

Most straightened styles depend on regular use of a hot comb together with what's called pressing oil. You should never use a hot comb on hair that has already been chemically straightened in a beauty parlor (details on straightening are in Chapter 10). This combination of heat and chemicals is just too much punishment for the hair to withstand. If your technique is good, you can use the hot comb at home. Beware, this is dangerous. It's merely a matter of applying pressing oil, then combing the hair with the electrically heated hot comb. The only potential danger is the chance of overheating the oil. Overly hot oil can slide down the hair shaft right into the follicle and cause a hair-loss condition called *hot-comb alopecia*. If the oil is hot enough, it can actually kill the follicle permanently. As such it represents one of the few mortal threats that ever imperil hair follicles.

All pressing oils and pressing creams are similar and widely available. The key thing to remember, besides carefully watching the heat, is that the hair must be *thoroughly rinsed and dried* before applying the oil. **Posner Pressing Oil Glossine** is a good product, as are **Gloss** and **Apex**, to name just a few.

Braids and corn rows can look great on some people, but they inevitably carry with them the danger of traction alopecia. Once in a while is okay. But never leave corn rows in for more than two days. Incidentally, corn rowing your hair will not make it grow faster.

Finally, a word on the Afro, which is not nearly so natural as it seems. To look good, Afro hairstyles require constant attention. The hair must be unceasingly trimmed, combed, and conditioned. About the worst thing you can do is to rake a metal Afro pick through a matted Afro. You might as well comb your hair with scissors! You'll get much better results if you wet the fingers with water or with water plus a little grooming oil, and first pull the hair into shape. Then comb it with a wide-spaced, blunt-toothed comb. Interestingly, the comb was invented in Africa. Not so the pick!

TYPICAL BLACK HAIR PROBLEMS

Many of the sufferers of a multisyllabic condition called *pseudofolliculitis* are black. Although it's not exclusive among blacks, it is related to the way most black hair grows. In pseudofolliculitis the hair is so curly that as it grows it pushes its own end right back into the follicle, producing what's called a "foreign-body reaction." White blood cells swarm to the area, resulting in bumps and pustules that look a lot like acne.

You can get pseudofolliculitis anywhere you have hair—on the scalp, pubis, underarms, etc. Shaving definitely can make it worse, either by irritating existing pustules or sharpening new hairs. The best treatment is daily preventive shampooing and combing to free up the hairs and keep them away from the skin surface. If you've already got it, then shampooing with an antibiotic shampoo like **Betadine** will soothe the infection while you free up your hair. In more serious cases you may need a doctor's prescription for a stronger antibiotic, such as tetracycline.

Pseudofolliculitis will usually go away with proper treatment. Not so *acne keloidalis of the scalp*. This is essentially the same condition except that it results in permanent thick scars called keloids instead of just temporary pustules. Sometimes the irritation of the ingrowing hair looks like advanced acne. If it gets really bad and cysts and pustules become seriously inflamed, then the accompanying masses of white blood cells can sometimes destroy the walls of the hair follicle. When it gets to this point, the condition is called *permanent*. There is simply no excuse for abusing your hair to this degree. See your doctor.

8

Away with Body and Facial Hair

The key concept, as far as hair removal is concerned, is that there is no such thing as perfection. The many home products and salon services described in this chapter are all very effective, but don't expect any of them to remove unwanted hair completely *forever*. That degree of perfection is just not possible. Whether or not you have too much hair in the wrong places is usually a personal aesthetic judgment. However, there are certain medical conditions that cause unwanted hair.

Too much hair stemming from medical reasons is called either *hirsutism* or *hypertrichosis*. The meanings of these terms actually overlap a bit, but they both refer to excessive hair on the face and/or body. Hirsutism is usually associated with women and children who have unusual amounts of body hair distributed in patterns similar to those of an adult male. This boils down to varying amounts of hair on arms, legs, cheeks, chin, upper lip, chest.

Hirsutism is occasionally a symptom of a serious neurological disease such as multiple sclerosis or meningitis. It can also accompany more general disorders, such as malnutrition,

certain cancers, even the mumps. Sometimes it's an indication of falling levels of estrogen, so that secondary male sex
characteristics such as facial hair can no longer be sup-
pressed. Or it can stem from a hormonal imbalance induced
by a course of new birth-control pills.

Hypertrichosis is the name for localized hair patches.
These can appear anywhere on the body and usually are
caused by some kind of trauma to the skin. Perhaps you've
seen or heard of the phenomenon of the bad burn that heals
and then grows a thick little pelt of hair. It's not uncommon.
Hypertrichosis can also be caused by any continual low-level
traumatization. For example, unwanted and unexpected hair
can spring up on skin that's been under a cast; it can grow
on the arms and legs of nervous people who ceaselessly
scratch and rub themselves; it can develop on the shoulders
of Third World peasants who spend their lives lugging
burlap sacks. Birthmarks and moles can also grow hair, as
can areas where hormone creams, particularly those containing steroids, have been continually applied for other medical
reasons.

Chronic thrombophlebitis, a disease in the news during the
Watergate years, can also cause hypertrichosis on the legs.
And then there's *hypertrichosis languinosa*, perhaps the most
sinister instance of too much hair. This condition, which
usually occurs in women, is marked by the sudden appearance of an eerily beautiful full white beard. It's quite
rare, which is fortunate, because it heralds the appearance of
a serious internal cancer.

Having said all this about the medical causes of hirsutism
and hypertrichosis, I now want to assure you that 99.9
percent of all cases of excess body hair are perfectly normal.
Far from being a symptom of a medical disorder, excess hair
is nearly always the result of a person's genetic recipe.
Parents with lots of body hair pass the genes along to their
children. Some people perceive their body hair as something
to get rid of, whereas others couldn't care less.

There are three basic approaches, or modalities, for hair removal: 1) electrical, 2) physical, and 3) chemical. Below is a discussion of each.

ELECTRICAL MODALITIES

Say "hair removal" and most people think of electrolysis. This is a time-tested technique that involves electrically frying the hair follicle in one of two ways.

The first type of electrolysis is performed with what's called direct galvanic current. It's the slower of the two methods, but it's usually more effective against regrowth. The other type is called electrocoagulation and involves a modified high-frequency electrical current. This method takes less time in the salon but has a higher incidence of regrowth.

Both methods involve the insertion of a fine wire needle into the opening of the hair follicle, followed by a little pinprick electrical shock. The electrical current, be it direct galvanic or modified high frequency, electrocutes and destroys the follicle. Or at least it's supposed to.

The degree of effectiveness depends considerably more on the competence of the operator than it does on the type of current employed. The same can be said for the safety factor. There's generally not much risk involved with electrolysis. However, a clumsy operator not only can make you very uncomfortable but can cause cuts that may leave small scars or cause small dark blotches called *hyperpigmentation*. The best way to find a competent electrolysis operator is to get a personal recommendation. If you don't have a friend who's had it done, ask your doctor if he or she can suggest someone.

Even with a good operator the process is tedious, expensive, and never complete. The American Medical Association estimates that a 40–60 percent rate of regrowth on treated areas is *normal.* This isn't because of bad operators. Some hairs will usually be below skin level during any electrolysis treatment, so their follicles won't be treated. And some sturdy follicles will simply not be destroyed by the electrical current.

People with lots of unattractive hair have to undergo weekly electrolysis treatments for three or four years. Even extensive treatment like this can't really grapple with large areas, such as arms or legs. Electrolysis is really for small areas on the face, the breasts, occasionally portions of the thighs or pubis. Large areas with lots of hair require different modalities. You'll have to trust the electrolysis operator if he or she tells you that the method isn't applicable to your hair problem.

There are also home electrolysis products called epilators. These are battery-operated appliances with a barrel handle from which extends a long wire needle that conducts current into the follicle. **Perma-Tweez** is a well-known brand that's mostly sold by mail order. It requires some practice to become good with these things. But if you do, the dollar savings over salon electrolysis visits can be considerable. You can find out about Perma-Tweez by writing to General Medical Co., 1935 Armacost Avenue, West Los Angeles, California 90025.

Recently there's been big news in hair removal, the arrival of **Depilatron**. This is a franchise operation and it's rapidly spreading. Depilatron probably destroys hair follicles by means of ultrasonic waves, just as a microwave oven cooks food. Because there's no shock, it's practically painless. And because it's considerably more comfortable than traditional electrolysis, a larger area can be treated in a sitting.

But, again, it's not perfect. The same percentage of hair grows back as would after traditional electrolysis. And it's similarly expensive. Even though it's faster than electrolysis, it's not fast enough to cope with large areas and lots of hair.

Again, it's mainly for small areas, usually on the face, and only occasionally elsewhere.

PHYSICAL MODALITIES

Hairs treated by electrolysis are easily plucked from the fried follicles. But the physical modalities we'll talk about here are primarily a matter of forcibly yanking hairs out while leaving the follicle alone completely.

The predominant hair-pulling method is waxing. It involves spreading hot wax onto the skin, allowing it to dry with the hairs embedded, then ripping it off. This is uncomfortable, true, but it's not so bad as it sounds. It leaves the skin surface free of hair, but of course makes no pretense of preventing or even of slowing down future growth.

You can usually have waxing done at the same places that offer electrolysis. Everybody gives his wax a little extra exotic touch. Some extol its purity; others claim it contains hormones like estrogen; still others embed a cloth in the wax which supposedly makes it easier to remove. I have yet to hear of an extra touch that really helped much. Again, the effectiveness rests largely on the competence of the person who does the waxing.

Waxing is for removing unwanted hair on large areas— waist, torso, legs, arms, back. It's much less expensive than any of the electrical modalities. What's more, you can easily do it at home with any of the wax hair removers sold in drugstores. **Zip Depilatory** is a good one. Like the others, it consists of a little tub of wax and simple directions on how to prepare the skin, melt and apply the wax, and how to yank it off. The wax is nonirritating, so you won't even have to do a sensitivity test.

Another common physical method is tweezing or plucking. You'll be glad to know that plucking your eyebrows will not make them grow back thicker or coarser. This goes for any plucked hair. If the hair is resting in a telogen follicle, then the plucking will probably flip the follicle back into the anagen growth phase. But the new hair that grows will not be any tougher than the one you plucked.

Similarly, shaving will not cause hairs to grow back either more thickly or more coarsely. The misconception about regrowth after shaving is as deeply embedded in the public consciousness as the erroneous connection of chocolate and acne. Doctors like myself can point to tests and experiments all day, and people still won't be convinced. Well, chocolate doesn't cause acne, and shaving doesn't cause coarsening hair regrowth.

Shaving can, however, cause painful and/or slow-healing nicks and cuts. I strongly urge people who shave their legs and underarms to use a fresh blade every time. The new disposable razors are admirably suited. Since the water-soaked hair is easier to cut, be sure to bathe or shower before shaving. Use a mild shaving cream, such as plain **Noxema**, which helps soothe minor irritations. Shave against the grain, and use long, even strokes.

Diabetics or women with varicose veins are liable to bad irritation stemming from razor nicks. These can look worse than unshaved legs. Whether or not you fall into either of these categories, I would strongly recommend an electric razor over a blade. When used with a preshave lotion, such as **Williams 'Lectric Shave**, you can get a smooth shave and effectively eliminate the chance of nicks, cuts, or razor burn.

Shaving is an effective—albeit short-term—solution to unwanted hair anywhere on the body. About the only place for potential trouble is in the vicinity of the pubis. The combination of sensitive skin and the sharp edge of a newly shaved and naturally curly terminal hair can easily lead to uncomfortable ingrown pubic hairs.

Finally, we come to the idea that what you can't see doesn't matter. That's the concept behind bleaching creams. **Jolen** and **Aime** are two good examples, both widely available. These products are easy to apply and come with simple directions. They usually tell you to clean the skin with cold water and soap, mix the cream with an accelerator that comes in the same package, then spread the mixture with a wooden spatula, also included in the kit. In this way you can treat arms, upper lip, brow, anywhere.

CHEMICAL MODALITIES

Both the desire for and the use of depilatories date back literally thousands of years B.C. One ancient recipe, preserved on papyrus scrolls, records ingredients that include burned tortoiseshell, malachite, hippo fat, plus a concoction of blood from oxen, goats, pigs, and dogs.

There's a lot that's right with today's chemical depilatories. They're cheap, safe, widely available, and effective. The number of people who are irritated or who have allergic reactions is minimal. The products have different formulas, but they're all based on the same active ingredient: thioglycolic acid. This remarkable substance is spread onto the hairy area, and it proceeds to soften and dissolve the hairs without harming the skin. After five to fifteen minutes—depending on the coarseness of the hair being removed—it can be wiped or washed away, leaving smooth skin behind. The best seller is **Nair**, but others in the field that are equally good include **Neet, Sleek, Surgex** (used by hospitals to prep surgical patients), **Nudit, Bu-To, Shimmy Shins.**

DR. ZIZMOR'S GUIDELINE CHART
FOR HAIR REMOVAL

With the following chart you can tell at a glance the recommended approaches for hair removal on various parts of the body.

Body Area	What You Can Do at Home	What You Can Have Done Professionally
face	epilators bleaching plucking shaving depilatories	electrolysis Depilatron
arms	bleaching waxing depilatories	waxing
legs	shaving depilatories waxing	waxing
pubis	epilators shaving	waxing
breast	shaving epilators	electrolysis Depilatron

9

Hair Coloring

As we go through life, our hair color naturally changes. This is as much a result of environment as aging. In fact, environment can literally wreak premature ruin on beautiful hair. For example, if you shampoo and blow dry too frequently, your lustrous mane can become dull and mousy; a shoddy or excessively calorie-restrictive diet can turn shining auburn hair drab and lusterless; too much ultraviolet light from sun exposure can turn fine blond hair into an over-bleached, unruly haystack. These are all natural enough occurrences, and they are described scientifically in what's called the *Evolutionary Hypothesis,* which posits that human hair color actually adapts to its environment. Summer lightening and winter darkening hark back to primitive prehumans who literally depended for their lives on protective coloring that blended with their changing surroundings.

Often environment alone is all that's causing an unsatisfactory hair color. In cases like this you're better off using a grooming product that's appropriate for your hair type (see Chapter 6) and not bothering at all trying to change your natural color.

Every human hair would be white as snow if it did not contain *melanin*. Like keratin, this is a protein produced inside the hair follicle. Melanin is capable of producing every hair color from platinum blond to Afro black. The exception that proves the rule is *phaeomelanin*, a close cousin responsible for redheads. Your personal hair color depends on two *genetically determined* factors: 1) the exact structure of your melanin proteins and 2) the exact location of the natural air bubbles in your hair shafts.

The infinite combinations of these two factors produce the wide spectrum of hair colors.

GRAYING

Gray hair is a normal sign of aging that typically make its debut by the beginning of the fourth decade of life. But you may carry an inherited gene that will cause a premature drop in your body's level of melanin production. In that case you'll be prematurely gray. The first gray usually starts at the temples, then spreads in thin waves to the crown, then finally to the neck. Various controversies surround the actual process of turning gray, but they all boil down to the same thing: lack of or change in melanin.

The difference in degree and shades of grayness is caused by two major factors. The first is the amount of still normally colored hairs intermixed with those turning gray. Remember that each hair follicle is like a ship on the sea. The cessation of melanin production in one follicle does not mean it won't be produced in adjacent follicles. There's also the matter of how light looks when it strikes the hair. This is a matter of the genetically determined structure of the hair shaft, specifically the location of air spaces. You can check two heads of hair with the same melanin structure and find that one can look silvery and the other dull gray depending on the reflection and refraction of light.

Graying hair is totally unrelated to hair loss. Neither does advancing grayness result in any other changes in the hair structure. If gray hair sometimes feels more coarse, it's only because of increasing dryness from the natural decline of scalp-oil secretions that accompanies aging.

Certain people suffer from medical conditions that include grayness as a symptom. A good example is *pernicious anemia*, the lack of vitamin B-12. In addition to grayness, anemia sufferers have a sour lemon-yellow complexion. Both the complexion and the grayness problems can be reversed with doses of B-12. Then there's thyroid disease. Whether you're *hyperthyroid* or *hypothyroid*, your hair can still turn prematurely gray. The same applies to sufferers of a complicated condition called *alopecia areata*. Usually because of some traumatic event, the hair can fall out either in patches or completely. When it comes back, it may grow in white. "Going white overnight" is an expression that describes severe and total alopecia areata. These people become so traumatized that all their hair falls out, usually over a day or two, and then grows back white. However, the hair color will eventually return. All these conditions, obviously, require professional attention.

There is no medical reason not to change the color of your hair. I say this notwithstanding the periodically announced carcinogenicity of various coloring agents. The superficial nature of hair-coloring procedures makes any threat of cancer from hair coloring too remote to be seriously considered. If changing your hair color makes you feel better, then go ahead and do it. Of course, hair color won't change your life, nor will it make you what you aren't. And if it's a matter of getting rid of gray, perhaps you should ask yourself if you don't really look more attractive *with* the gray.

SHOULD YOU OR SHOULDN'T YOU?
A HISTORICAL PERSPECTIVE

Hair coloring and bleaching date back to antiquity. The Egyptian queen Sess is credited with having started the craze for henna thousands of years ago. Henna is a totally organic, plant-derived semipermanent dye that is as effective today as it was thousands of years ago. It was revived in the nineteenth century by a famous Italian singer named Adelina Patti. Her hair was an astonishing reddish-purple color, and when she toured America in 1859, it caused a sensation.

The fashion craze for henna came on the heels of the declining popularity of bleaching. The lust for lighter hair is said to have originated among patrician Roman ladies. They were thunderstruck by the golden tresses of prisoners brought from Northern Europe by the Roman legions. It didn't take long for the fashion-conscious Romans to devise special concoctions to bleach the hair at least to a golden redness, if not quite to Viking blondness.

The bleaches of ancient Rome were not particularly therapeutic for the hair. Made from rock alum, quicklime, wood ash, and lots of old wine, they often left hair pretty damaged. Still, this basic formula remained in use until well into the Middle Ages.

Interestingly enough, the first soap made in Europe was prepared not for the purpose of washing but to bleach the hair. Made from goat fat, these "Mattiac balls"—sometimes Gaul was called Mattiac—represented a major improvement over the old Roman process. Still, the Mattiac balls left much to be desired, and, in retrospect, the people would doubtless have been better off using them for bathing (an almost unheard-of practice in medieval Europe).

By the sixteenth century the Renaissance was in full swing in Southern Europe, and painters such as Titian and Botticelli were making golden-blond tresses newly fashionable. Since the first appearance of Mattiac balls people had been experimenting with all kinds of combinations of alum, ashes, borax, birch bark, saffron, myrrh, and the ubiquitous old wine. But in Renaissance Venice they came up with the most effective formula yet, a combination of soda, black sulfur, and honey. This concoction, which was spread on the hair and allowed to dry in the sun, remained the treatment of choice for centuries. It wasn't until the time of Adelina Patti that bleaching went into a temporary eclipse, and all these damaging and unreliable treatments were generally discontinued.

It's only been in the last fifty years that bleaching has been perfected, because of the advent of *hydrogen peroxide,* which is relatively safe, effective, cheap, and even critical to the effectiveness of coloring dyes.

Hydrogen peroxide has a remarkable reaction to keratin, causing both physical and chemical changes. On the physical level, it opens the imbrications of the cuticle just enough to be able to penetrate the hair shaft without causing significant damage. Once inside, it chemically changes the melanin coloring proteins by means of oxidation. Yes, it's the same hydrogen peroxide that's sold in drugstores as a disinfectant. Only the variety used on hair is significantly more concentrated.

WAYS TO CHANGE YOUR HAIR COLOR

You can either have your hair color changed professionally, or you can do it yourself. Either way, the basic steps and the preparations employed are essentially the same. It might be a good idea to go to a salon for your first hair-coloring job and take the opportunity to observe closely the proper technique. The only thing a salon can give you that you can't give yourself is the benefit of being treated by a colorist with experience. But coloring knowledgeability is not really all that esoteric, and you *can* pick it up yourself.

There are three basic approaches to changing the color of the hair. The first involves simply using a hydrogen-peroxide bleaching solution, such as **Clairol's Clairoxide**, to lighten the hair. The second involves using hydrogen peroxide together with either a synthetic or an organic hair dye. Major manufacturers make these dyes in every conceivable color. On the Roux color chart, by way of example, you can find everything from Chocolate Kiss to Tempting Taffy. L'Oréal, Revlon, Clairol, and all the other big manufacturers offer a similarly large choice of colors. The third approach includes miscellaneous coloring agents that are not used with hydrogen peroxide. These include temporary washable dyes, semipermanent dyes, henna, certain metallic dyes.

About the only medically chancy aspect of coloring your hair is a potential allergic reaction to some dyes. At times it's not even the dye but the perfume or the peroxide or something else. Since hair coloring involves a number of ingredients, there's always a chance that you may be the one in the multitude who's allergic to one of them.

Although uncommon, these allergic reactions can really turn into a problem. The eruptions they cause are called *contact dermatitis*. This condition can make you look as though you have poison ivy—redness, oozing, crusting, and blistering. Some people are fooled because the eruption usually takes twenty-four to forty-eight hours. And then, instead of affecting the scalp where the dye was applied, it usually occurs on the neck and/or forehead, probably because the irritating agent is often shampooed thoroughly out of the hair but not so thoroughly off the neck and forehead.

The appearance of these delayed hypersensitive reactions is well understood by every manufacturer of permanent and semipermanent hair-coloring products, so their products include instructions on how to give yourself a sensitivity test. The test involves mixing a small amount of the ingredients and applying them to the inner fold of your elbow, letting them dry for a day, then watching for another day to see if anything develops. Usually nothing will. If it does, you should not, of course, use that product all over your head. Beauty salons are supposed to give you the same test, but many of them probably don't allow enough time to pass to tell if you're really allergic or not.

Some final thoughts on allergic reactions to hair dye:

1. Just because you've been using a color for years and years doesn't mean you can't develop a sudden allergy to it. *Sensitization*, or the process of becoming allergic, can be gradual, sometimes taking many years. That's why you must do a patch test every time before you dye.

2. Because of the inexorable process of gradual sensitization, all manufacturers regularly change their formulas ever so slightly just to be sure no one uses enough to become sensitized. However, this is unfortunate for those few individuals who will demonstrate allergic reactions to the new ingredient(s) in the changed formula.

3. There's also the government to consider. Carcinogens, which is the name for agents linked to cancer, are being exposed every day. No matter if a laboratory rat would have to dye its hair daily a thousand times for a thousand years with carbon black #1, if the dye gave the rat a tumor in the lab, off the market it comes. Whenever the government orders something off the market, manufacturers have to substitute it with something else. And sometimes that something will give you an unexpected allergic reaction.

Even if you do have an allergic reaction to a hair-coloring product, it usually goes away in a relatively short time. More importantly, your new color, once it's fixed on the hair, will not keep on irritating. Even if a rash appears well before twenty-four hours have elapsed, you can wash your hair with a mild shampoo like **Johnson's Baby Shampoo** and rid yourself of the irritating agents.

Applications of cool compresses soothe these rashes, just as they soothe poison ivy. You can make a good compress by filling a quart bottle with crushed ice and adding a heaping tablespoon of salt and a cup of milk. The measures don't have to be exact, and the compresses, which you can make from any handy cotton or linen cloth, don't have to be sterile. Shake the compress mixture and apply the wet cloth to the affected area three to four times daily for periods of fifteen minutes.

SIMPLE BLEACHING

Plain hydrogen-peroxide bleach is what you'll use if you only want to lighten your hair without adding any coloring agent. All you have to do is put it on, wait, and wash it out, although a visit to a beauty salon is helpful in learning the most efficient way to part the hair and apply the solution.

The amount of time you let the solution stay on the hair determines how light the hair becomes. In order to test for desired color, most products recommend that you apply the peroxide solution to a small swatch of hair at the same time you do your sensitivity test. In this way you can get two birds with one stone, testing how long you'll have to keep the solution on the hair while testing for any reaction on the skin.

Good permanent bleaches that contain peroxide and conditioners but no coloring dyes include **Born Blond Lightener, Summer Blond**, and **Lemon Go Lightly**, all by Clairol, and **Ultra Silk Hair Lightener** and **Snow Silk Lightener** by Revlon. You can also lighten already blond hair by using a gentle peroxide lightener in conjunction with sunlight or a sunlamp. Good products include **Clairol's Lemon Go Lightly** and **Midnight Sun, Sun-In** by Gillette, and **Young Blond** by L'Oréal. (By the way, lemon juice is *not* a bleaching agent— even in the sun.)

FROSTING, TIPPING, STREAKING AND HAIR PAINTING

The primary advantage of these techniques is that they don't have to be repeated so frequently to continue to look good. And although they employ peroxide bleach, the bleach doesn't get on the scalp, which automatically reduces the chance of allergic reaction on the skin.

Frosting achieves an overall salt-and-pepper effect that can look attractive. It's most frequently done with a perforated rubber cap, through which perforations the individual strands of hair are pulled. Only those hairs are bleached, and the others are left the natural color.

Tipping is similar except that clusters of hairs are bleached together, and the bleach solution is applied from a point about half inch above the scalp. The clumps of bleached hair are often wrapped in tin foil while the bleach solution is working.

Streaking is a technique designed to achieve drama, a la Gloria Steinem. Again, it's just selective bleaching, and the success of the effect depends on the compatibility of your natural hair color plus the artistry of the application.

Finally, there's hair painting, which is streaking with a brush. Whether or not it looks good depends on the applier's technique. You can buy hair-painting kits, but it would seem a prudent idea to have it done professionally the first time, unless you're very sure of yourself.

Peroxide frosting and tipping dyes are widely available. **Clairol's Frost and Tip** is good; so are the **Quiet Touch Hair Painting Kit** and **Summer Blond**.

All bleaching carries with it the possibility of harsh-

looking hair tone. This is especially the case with intense
highlighting techniques. To soften the harshness, you should
use a toner, such as **Revlon's Blond Silk, Clairol's Born Blond
Lotion Toner, L'Oréal Preference Perfect Blond,** or **Revlon's
Color Silk Crystal Lights,** to name only a few.

PERMANENT DYES USED WITH PEROXIDE

Permanent dyes used in combination with separately bottled peroxide are all similar in concept to bleaches. You have
to do a sensitivity patch test, then a swatch test to determine
how much time is necessary to achieve desired color. No
matter what you use, you'll be warned to keep it out of your
eyes on pain of possible blindness. And you can't store dye-
peroxide mixture, since it has a tendency to explode when
left sealed for too long.

It used to be that all the elements for permanently
coloring the hair had to be purchased separately. Of course,
you can still do it that way, in which case you'll have to buy
the dye in whatever shade you choose, the peroxide (usually
called a developer), an applicator bottle, and plastic gloves.
Fortunately, you can also buy boxed hair-color sets that
include everything. Be sure you know what you're getting.
Some women buy hair dye and don't realize until they get
home that they need a half dozen other things.

Clairol's Nice'n Easy line and **L'Oréal's Preference** series
are two examples of completely packaged hair-coloring kits.
The boxes contain everything you'll need, right down to the
plastic gloves. They also contain rather forbiddingly long
instruction sheets, which you absolutely must study. But
having read this chapter, you won't find the instructions so
complicated.

The use of peroxide with color dyes rests on its ability to
open imbrications of the cuticle and allow the dyes to get
into the hair shaft. Dye-developer mixtures are applied in a

variety of ways. Some products go on as a shampoo; others are just poured onto the head and allowed to sit quietly for the predetermined time limit. The dyeing phase is always followed by a thorough shampoo to stop the coloring process.

Every company makes a wide selection of hair colors. Sometimes they even seem to be competing with themselves. The point of it all, presumably, is to get you to experiment. Good color dye lines include **Breck Hair Color, Clairol Balsam Color, Color Silk** by Revlon, **European Naturals** by Alberto-Culver, **Excellence Extra Rich Hair Color** by L'Oréal, **Fanci-Tone** by Roux, **Miss Clairol Hair Color Bath Creme Formula, Tried and True** by Max Factor, **Preference** by L'Oréal, **Clairol's Nice 'n Easy**, and many others.

Hair dyes are strong, and the colors bind organically and permanently to the hair. It's imperative to wait at least three to four weeks between colorings, or you might weaken the hair. If you decide your new color is a mistake or that you've put in too much, relax. Dye manufacturers make safe dye solvents. Good ones include **Delete** by Roux, **Effasol** by L'Oréal, and two others made by Clairol, called, respectively, **Metalex** and **Remov-zit.**

All colors, be they natural or chemically induced by dyes, will oxidize to some extent. Usually hair is cut off before it has a chance to show much noticeable oxidation. Occasionally the natural lightening of oxidation is perceived in reddening. There is no standard rate of hair oxidation; it varies from head to head. If your dyed hair seems to be reddening, you can either use more dye or try another product which may resist oxidation better on your hair.

HAIR COLORING WITHOUT PEROXIDE

There's a whole category of temporary hair dyes that wash out with a single shampoo. These products coat only the cuticle and often have a shine-inducing acid pH. In fact, their major advantage lies in their noninterference with cuticle imbrications. They also come in many colors and rarely require time-consuming allergy-pat 4 or color-swatch tests.

On the other hand, they tend to rub off on pillows and clothing, and will actually wash out should you be caught in a rainstorm. They must be reapplied after every shampoo, which is inconvenient and may cause dullness buildup.

What's more, these colors can be used only to *darken* the hair.

There are many temporary hair-color products, and the following list hardly includes everything. These, however, are all good: **Come Alive Gray** by Clairol, **Picture Perfect Color Rinse** by Clairol, **Fanci-Full Rinse** by Roux, **Nestlé Protein Color Rinse**, **Noreen Color Hair Rinse**, **Streaks 'n Tips** by Nestlé.

The next category is the semipermanent dyes. This group of products also works without benefit of peroxide; instead it combines vegetable dyes with chemicals such as sulfur and anomium thioglycolate.

Semipermanent hair colors have advantages midway between the temporaries and the permanents. They last through more than one shampoo, but they will fade and wash out in a month or so. They won't rub off so easily, but they do require the same patch and swatch tests used with permanent dyes. On balance, they are relatively easy to use, require no mixing of dyes and developers, and, compared to permanent dyes, they don't react so strongly with the hair shaft.

Here is a short list of good semipermanent color lines: **Happiness** by Clairol, **Loving Care Color Foam** by Clairol, **Loving Care Hair Color Lotion** by Clairol, **Silk and Silver Color Lotion, Touch of Silver** by L'Oréal.

Next we have the so-called hair restorers. These don't change your hair color but, rather, restore your original color gradually. They do it with metallic dyes and salts of various metals, such as silver, copper, manganese, cobalt. **Lady Grecian Formula, RD,** and **Youthair** are good examples. You comb them through the hair after every shampoo, and gradually the hair darkens and the gray vanishes.

Finally, there's **henna**, a harmless, nonirritating permanent dye that's been around for thousands of years. Henna, manufactured today by a company called Hopkins, comes from the leaves of an African bush. It's mixed in a bowl and applied to the hair either as a rinse or a paste. Henna now comes in a variety of shades, but they *all* fall into the red-to-auburn part of the spectrum. Depending on how long you leave it on, it results in varying degrees of reddish highlights. Except for occasional buildup problems, henna works very well.

10

Waving and Straightening

From the standpoint of a strand of hair, waving and straightening are the same thing. In either case the hair undergoes the same three stages. First, you soften the hair; second, you rearrange the softened hair into a new position; finally, you chemically halt the reaction period with a special neutralizer, after which the hair will retain its new alignments.

The chemicals used in home-permanent products do not vary from the professional-salon products. But a good stylist has plenty of experience and won't make the same mistakes you will, especially if you're trying something for the first time. If you're contemplating your first permanent, my advice definitely would be to go to a professional. See it done well the first time, because you'll be able to do almost as well yourself at home once you get a good rolling-and-timing technique.

Hair waving as a salon treatment made its debut in nineteenth-century Europe. The term "marcelled" derives from the name Marcel Grateau, the man who first used heat to curl the hair. He did this by wrapping it around hot irons. The results, however, were only temporary. A German chemist named Julius Nessler is credited with being the first to create permanent curls by combining heat with chemicals. He used hot spools, together with pads soaked in an alkali solution closely related to ammonia. Combined with heat, the alkali effectively opened the imbrications and allowed the hair to accept fully the new curled position.

At first this method was used only on wigs, but it soon became a fashion rage despite its considerable shortcomings. The heated spools were heavy and sometimes got too hot. If they didn't scorch the scalp, they often baked the alkali pads right onto the hair. The trend-setting women of the day suffered this not only with forbearance but apparently with relish. The torture one underwent for stylish curls was actually the subject of drawing-room chatter of the most fashionable sort.

WAVING YOUR HAIR

The easiest and safest way to wave the hair is with a water wave, which involves nothing more than letting freshly washed hair dry on rollers. It causes a temporary, cohesive set that usually lasts for a day but disappears the minute your hair gets wet.

Large rollers make large, casual waves; small rollers make tight little waves. Hair dries faster on wire-mesh curlers, but curls look smoother if you use smooth plastic rollers. Heat, either from a blow dryer or from electric curlers, will enhance the curling, since it tends to soften the hair slightly.

Water waves are stronger and last longer if a setting lotion is applied to the hair while it's wet and on the curlers. Setting lotions, which also come in gel form, contain the same hair lacquers and plasticizers found in aerosol hair sprays. They'll hold a curl only until it gets wet.

Chemical waving is a different story. With this method you get permanent curls that last—at least to some degree—until the hair is cut off. These curls relax slightly in the course of months of normal washing and brushing. But the stronger the hair shaft, the better it can accept and hold the chemically induced curl.

Salon permanents often use intense heat; home permanents rarely do. There is no doubt that heating rolled hair that's been treated with a chemical wave solution will impart a stronger curl than just letting the solution sit on the hair at room temperature. So if experience is the most valuable thing a salon can offer you, then strong heat for your curlers is certainly the second most important.

But even without heat you certainly can give yourself an effective permanent at home. You just can't get it quite so curly. As a matter of fact, the development of the postwar "machineless" cold wave truly revolutionized the beauty business. It introduced permanent waving into the home, where it has been flourishing for decades. Today you can buy entire home permanent kits that contain 1) a waving solution, 2) a hydrogen-peroxide neutralizer to stop the waving action, and 3) highly detailed instructions on use.

Almost anybody can curl hair at home unless the hair is very fine. How well the hair holds a curl depends on the diameter of the hair shaft and the proportion of cortex to cuticle.

The cortex holds the wave, not the cuticle. Proportionately, there is less cortex on a shaft of fine hair than on a similar shaft of coarse hair. Coarse hair, with its thicker diameter, better withstands the strain of chemical softening and rehardening. And its thicker cortex holds the wave better. The slimmer cortex of fine hair tends either to hold the wave poorly or to break during the waving process.

The active ingredient in most permanent-wave solutions is

thioglycolate. This is the same ingredient contained in chemical depilatories like Nair. Thioglycolates soften the hair and disrupt its natural chemical bonds. The softened hair then accepts its curled position on the roller, after which the head is rinsed with water and a chemical neutralizer. The rinse is naturally done well before the thioglycolate has a chance to soften the hair too much. Usually the neutralizer is some sort of hydrogen-peroxide solution that chemically reverses the thioglycolate effect and rehardens the hair.

Problem reactions to home hair permanents are fairly common. Sometimes you can make your hair brittle and filled with split ends, and occasionally undue amounts of hair will break off at the scalp. These reactions are usually caused either by leaving the chemicals on too long or by improper neutralization. The split ends can be helped with conditioners but cured only by cutting them off. As for the fragile and broken hair, you may take some small comfort from the knowledge that the follicles will still be able to grow new hair.

There are also people who have allergic reactions to some of the chemicals used in permanent waving. Fortunately, this happens rarely, but that's again small comfort if you're the one with the weeping, oozing red eruptions. Usually you can stop the irritation well before it becomes too serious by rinsing with cold water, applying the neutralizer, then rinsing thoroughly again. If it's really necessary, you can further soothe the irritated areas by applying cold compresses dipped in a solution made from a quart of cold water or melting crushed ice into which you've mixed a cup of skim milk and two tablespoons of salt.

At home the best insurance against these problems is to follow the package directions closely. No matter where you get your permanent, be sure your hair is strong enough to handle the process. If it's been recently and/or regularly

bleached or dyed, think twice before you bathe it in thioglycolate. It's okay to wave bleached or colored hair, but if
the hair is already dry, hard to manage, and/or brittle from
chemical treatments, then it's going to be much more liable
to damage from the waving chemicals.

Manufacturers of home permanents make special formulas
for hard- and easy-to-wave hair, and they also package their
products in gel and liquid form. They really do try hard to
make it easy, but home permanents occasionally fail. When
they do, it is almost always a case of not leaving the waving
solution on long enough or of not applying the neutralizer
properly. Without proper neutralizer to reharden the softened hair, it will simply return to its original straightness as
soon as the rollers are removed.

Hair should be well cut and freshly washed before a
permanent. The procedure is to comb strands of hair up from
the scalp, apply the permanent-wave solution, wind the
strand onto a roller, and clip. When heat is used, endpapers
are wrapped over the end of each strand of hair to prevent
crushing of the hair ends while rolling up the strand.
Without heat the crushing doesn't matter and the endpapers
are optional. Don't try to put too large a strand of hair onto
any one roller, especially if your hair is thick. Roller placement is important. Keep the rollers close together, lest your
finished curls appear unattractively separated from one another. Make sure your rollers are rolled in the direction you
want the hair to curl. If you want body waves, then alternate
the direction of each row of rollers. Be sure that clips used
on pin curlers are rustproof and allow for easy drying.
There's no doubt that the best way to learn good roller
placement is to watch a professional do it.

After the neutralizing state of a home permanent there is a
way to add a little curl-enhancing heat yourself. Just dry the
rolled hair with a blow dryer, which will make your hair

curlier and your curls longer lasting. Since the hair doesn't fully set for twenty-four hours, be careful when you remove the rollers. Let those new curls cool fully before brushing them out. And brush the hair in the opposite direction from the way you rolled the curls, so as to minimize crimp marks on the scalp. You can also use a hair spray to help keep the curls tight for the first night, but don't use too much. Paradoxically, too much hair spray can make freshly permanented curls go limp. Probably the best idea is just to blow dry the hair or to let it dry naturally, then brush the curls out gently when they're completely cool.

What happens if you make your hair too curly? Don't worry. Since curls don't fully set for a day, you can easily relax them. **Clairol Condition** will do the job, as will **Metalex Conditioner and Corrective.**

Super Toni, the "Advance Look Perm," by Gillette; **Twin Conditioning Gentle Toni**, also by Gillette; and **Amino Organic Permanent Wave**, by Palm Beach Beauty Products, are three typical home-permanent kits that come complete with everything you'll need and with full instructions.

STRAIGHTENING YOUR HAIR

The simplest way to straighten long, wavy hair is to use your own head as a roller. Simply wash the hair and leave it wet, then wrap it around the head like a turban and fasten with clips. Use a large roller for the hair on the crown of the head. When the hair dries, dampen it again with plain water and wrap it around the head in the opposite direction. After the second drying, you can simply comb the straightened hair with a wide-toothed comb.

There are a few other simple physical modalities for straightening the hair. Hair dressings like **Alberto VO5** or

Clairol's Vitapointe are even easier than the head turban mentioned above. These greasy preparations hold the hair in place and are especially good for pulled-back hairstyles, in which the hair is worn close to the head. The only risk is of pores near the hairline becoming clogged with oil, which can lead to acne.

Another approach is to straighten the hair with heat. You can pull wet curls over a brush with one hand and train a blow dryer on the brush with the other. Many blowers have a special nozzle just for this. It works well, but it takes time and is very drying to the hair. It's certainly nothing you'd want to do every day.

You can also spread your hair on an ironing board and iron the curls out. This works, too, but you'll undoubtedly need a friend to help and a good-luck charm to avoid burning either the hair or the scalp. Keep the iron on the lowest end of the "warm" setting.

Another method is the electric hot comb, together with scented pressing oils, which act as a heat-transfer medium. This method has been around since the beginning of the twentieth century, and hot combs have now been perfected. The effect is only temporary, however. The hair stays straight only until it gets wet in the shower or moisturized on a wet or humid day. And there's a substantial risk that overly hot pressing oil will damage the hair follicles.

Chemical straighteners unquestionably do the best job, but they also carry the most risk. In addition to thioglycolates, there are two other chemical straightening families: sodium-hydroxide types, which are closely related to lye, and ammonium- or sodium-bisulfite lotions.

Thioglycolate straighteners are practically the same as the permanent-wave products mentioned earlier. You can apply them to clean, damp hair for varying lengths of time, from 10 to 15 minutes, then, instead of rolling the hair into curl-

setting spools, you comb it out for 20 minutes. After that you
rinse and apply the neutralizer. Here's a list of good thioglycolate products, each of which comes with full directions
and all the materials you'll need:

> **Curl-Away** by Continental Babs
> **Curls Away** by Richard Hudnut
> **Go Straight** by Nutritonic
> **Set Me Straight** by Rexall
> **Sudden Silk** by Evans
> **Wellastrate** by Wella
> **Straight Set** by Max Factor
> **Smooth Away** by Helene Curtis

Sodium-hydroxide straighteners are very strong alkaline
products that require extra-careful attention to instructions.
These straighteners are very effective, but they are more
likely to irritate skin and are dangerous if they get into the
eyes. On the other hand, they work faster by causing the hair
to swell rapidly and require half as much combing before the
neutralizer is applied. You can buy them as lotions or
creams, and here's a list of good ones:

> **Apex Natural Perm** by Apex
> **Ever Perm** by Helene Curtis
> **Hair Strate** by Summit Labs
> **Royal Crown Relaxer Permanent**
> **Ultra Wave** by Johnson & Johnson

Finally, we have the ammonium- or sodium-bisulfite
straighteners. These are the newest and safest of the chemical relaxers, but they're also, unfortunately, the least effective. For hair that's not extremely curly they're great. The
solutions are applied to clean, wet hair, then left on for 15

minutes under a plastic turban. After that the hair is combed for 20 minutes, then neutralized. Good products include the following:

Curlaxer by Posner
Curl Free by Gillette
U.N.C.U.R.L. by Clairol
Vege-Kurl

Part II
Hair Help from Professionals

11

Hairstyles and Professional Stylists

The cost of having your hair stylishly cut falls within a huge range. My feeling is as follows: Price means less if you go less. The cost of a good cut reflects both the talent of the person who does it and the popularity of the establishment in which he or she works. This cost is whatever the market will bear, typically higher in the big cities and lower in the suburban and outlying areas. In no event do low prices suggest cheaper materials; no reputable place uses them.

I recommend that anybody who lives in or near a big city go to the most famous hair salon in town—at least for the first cut. These places nearly always attract the area's most talented and original professionals to their staffs. If you're planning to change your look and get a new hairstyle, go to the best first. Local salons can always copy the high-priced cut later. Talented stylists have a flair for line and body, and they sell haircuts that last. They won't cast a woman's hair in plastic sprays, nor will they leave either sex with a style that vanishes without a trace after the first shampoo.

There is no reason for a good hairstyle not to be durable. Anyone can get theatrical results by working you over for half an hour with a blow dryer. But good stylists give haircuts that look good when they're wet, too. It's the shape that counts. And a well-shaped and styled head of hair makes invaluable contributions to your sense of well-being and attractiveness. It's worth the occasionally extravagant price.

Few people recognize or appreciate their own good points. Almost everybody hates his nose or thinks his forehead is too high or too low or too something. It takes a talented stylist, with a good artistic sense, to pick a style that makes both the hair and the face look good. A talented stylist will also give you a style that brings out your best points without obligating you to make more salon visits than you desire or can afford.

Before getting a state license to practice, stylists go to beautician school. The approaches they teach at beautician school are no longer universally accepted, and in fact many hair superstars have made their reputations by purposely breaking traditional beauty-school rules.

These rules rest on a basic assumption: the desirability of the "oval" face. If the client doesn't have an oval face, then the beauty school teaches the stylist to cut the hair in a manner that will make the face look oval. Rightly or wrongly, the oval is deemed the classic standard. In working with it, the stylist doesn't have to play down any of the features, and almost any hairstyle will look good.

If the face isn't oval, beauty schools and cosmetology textbooks° teach the following standard approaches:

1. *The diamond-shaped face.* This is a case of a narrow chin, wide cheekbones, and a narrow forehead. The task of the stylist is to give an oval look by flattening the diamond. This is done with a style that gives fullness on the forehead and the lower cheekbones and oftentimes includes bangs.

2. *The heart-shaped face.* This face has a narrow chin and

° A good one for the average reader is *Textbook of Cosmetology* by Oliver P. Scott (Prentice-Hall).

a wide forehead. So hair is combed onto the forehead to minimize the area, is kept close to the temples, and is flaired for a fuller look below.

3. *The square face.* This face has a wide jaw and an equally wide forehead. The traditional solution is to bring the hair forward and close to the face and to comb it off the forehead into framing curls.

4. *The oblong face.* This face is somewhat elongated and often sits on top of a long neck. The beauty-school approach is to get hair onto the forehead and to frame the rest of the face with waves to soften the natural angularity.

5. *The round face.* Here there's both a wide hairline and fullness in the lower face. Very often the real solution to a round face is for the customer to lose ten pounds. In lieu of that the stylist is traditionally advised to comb and tease height onto the top of the head.

6. *The pear-shaped face.* This is a case of a wide jaw surmounted by a small forehead. The standard approach is to add width and fullness at eye level and above the ears but to keep the hair close to the lower cheeks and nape of the neck.

Beauty-school students are also taught to consider the customer's profile. The three basic profile categories are straight (like Marilyn Monroe's); concave (like Popeye the Sailor's); and convex (like Barbra Streisand's). The profile influences the lines on which they style the rest of the head.

MODERN HAIRSTYLE DEVELOPMENTS

Mass hairstyles change slowly, and a really new style is a rarity. Actually, hair fashion comes close to being a measured alternation between so many years of long hair followed by so many years of short hair. These fashion cycles alternate almost as the stock market does. First comes a growth phase, usually triggered by trend-setting celebrities and socialites;

then comes the speculation, when every salon from city center to suburb to farming center offers the style or a modest variation thereof; finally comes the sell-off, when only the unfashionable outlanders continue to get the same hair-do, out of habit, while the trend setters are well into something new.

A really new style is usually a function of large-scale changes in life-style and technology. We saw this most recently in the late 1950s, when the short, layered cut made its debut. Before that most women wore their hair hidden under a hat. The Italian layered cut was short and it was put on rollers and sometimes blow dried for volume.

The volume was what really made it different. And as layer cutting gradually filtered down from Rome and Hollywood into neighborhood beauty parlors, the new concept of volume underwent successive, sometimes dubious, improvements. Hair began to go onto bigger and bigger rollers and eventually emerged as the bubble. Bangs appeared as standard equipment. Since many women couldn't or wouldn't cut their hair fast enough, bubbles began turning into bouffants. And at the extreme they evolved into the much-maligned beehive.

Besides blow dryers, the galloping technology of the postwar years also gave us realistic-looking and reasonably priced artificial hair. It wasn't long before falls were sharing space with huge beehives on the same impossible-to-maintain heads.

A more recent development is the razor cut, which has the same effect on the hair shaft as scissors. It is a technique used to achieve the so-called serf look. Where else would the serf look start but in high society? This cut is short in the front and longer in the back. It is still in the process of filtering through society, sometimes improved beyond recognition with various curls and bangs.

At the same time that some women are walking around with beehives others are paying no attention to any of this.

THE NINE CLASSIC HAIRSTYLES

Whether you realize it or not, whenever you go for a cut and a blowout your stylist is seeing your hairstyle as nothing more than a variation on one of the nine classic styles. If the stylist is good, then he'll give your hair an extra flattering shape and flair. But his basic vocabulary rests on these styles.

A word of advice: Give your stylist feedback both during and after the job. You don't have to take advice that strikes you as weird or impractical. If you don't like what you see, speak up before you get out of the chair. You can be flexible and open to suggestion without being railroaded into something your inner self tells you is all wrong.

The foremost American hair stylist, Kenneth, in his book *Kenneth's Complete Book on Hair* (Dell, 1972), lists nine "classic" hair styles. You may be well advised to try some of them in front of a mirror at home. It'll make your decisions easier when you arrive for your styling appointment.

1. *The french twist.* This style gives a look of neatness and tidiness. The hair is pulled back on both sides and fastened into a small, twisted bun that's worn at the crown.

2. *The chignon.* Ballerinas traditionally wear this particular style. It's essentially a French twist with a larger and more ornate bun at the crown.

3. *The ponytail.* This one is classic and easy. Beware of pulling the hair back too tightly, lest you induce traction alopecia (a temporary hair loss from pulling too hard on the hair).

4. *Long and swingy.* It looks great on college girls or on anyone with lustrously beautiful hair. The problem is really

one of maintenance. This style is liable to tangles, accumulations of dirt, and split ends.

5. *Short and curly.* The style is highly favored by women with office jobs. The curls are either natural or set on rollers.

6. *Short and straight.* By far the easiest of all to live with.

7. *All one length.* This is the classic American look; the hair frames the face, like Julie Christie's hairstyle in *Shampoo.*

8. *The pageboy.* This, you'll recall, is hair that's short in the front and long in the back and is also called the serf.

9. *The Afro.* Very curly hair worn in a soft, expanded halo. Looks good but requires lots of maintenance.

CHOOSING STYLES AND SALONS

The golden rule of hairstyling is "To thine own self be true." Don't get a style that falls down in two days if you can come to the beauty parlor only once every two months. Consider your life-style and try to picture your hairstyle as a part of it. Do you spend your days on a tennis court or over a washer-dryer, in front of an office typewriter or in the public library, on a tractor or in a board room? Do you have time to care for an intricate hairstyle, or are you constantly on the run from one thing to another?

I'm all for getting a new hairstyle if it'll make you more attractive. Life keeps going on; you change; your feelings change; your friends change; there's no reason not to change your hair, too. It's healthy, but by all means be practical.

It's a mistake to choose a hairstyle that contradicts your own image of yourself. High fashion is all well and good, and the girls in the pages of *Vogue* are certainly gorgeous. But if you think you might not feel comfortable with a certain fashionable haircut, then listen to yourself. Besides, beautiful as many of the magazine girls are, it takes *hours* to prepare them for a photo that takes a fraction of a second.

During your styling appointment be prepared to tell the stylist what you want. Don't leave it up to him to read your mind; and by the same token, don't be too single-minded to take his advice. Tell the stylist why you're there. Are you going to a wedding tomorrow, preparing for a week's work in the office, or about to leave for a summer in Europe? Be sure the stylist knows your sensitive points. If you have a scar, prominent bones, or anything else you want to divert attention from, let him or her know.

If there's a certain style you saw in a magazine or newspaper, tear it out and bring it along to the salon. Verbal descriptions can't compare to a photo of the real thing. Be sure your stylist knows how to give you that look; in big-name, big-city salons you can usually expect that they will. Finally, listen to the stylist's opinion of how the style will look on you. You're paying for his or her experience, so it's foolish not to pay attention to it. The stylist may point out compelling reasons why a particular style would look terrible on your head.

There's enough competition in the hairdressing market for you to be able to expect a pleasant atmosphere at any good cutting-and-styling salon. There's no need to tolerate coldness, lack of interest, or snobbery. I like an establishment that's owner-managed, one that welcomes customers hospitably and takes a personal interest in the way the hair comes out. Places like this usually respect the value of your time, too. They'll make an effort to get you an appointment when you need one, and they won't keep you waiting for an hour when you arrive.

A CHECKLIST TO RATE HAIRSTYLE SALONS

1. *Hours and location.* It's not practical to go to a place that's open only from nine to five if that's when you work. It's also nuts to try to squeeze an appointment in at noon or five o'clock. As a rule of thumb, you get less attention at peak hours. Sometimes—and particularly in the case of a famous and/or highly respected style salon—it's worth the inconvenience of a hard-to-get appointment to get that first superprofessional cut. But if you're looking for a place to patronize regularly, pick one that's convenient to your normal routine. Incidentally, a few years ago there was a twenty-four-hour beauty salon that opened in New York City. I thought it was a great idea, especially for career women. Interestingly, it was popular when it opened but eventually went out of business.

2. *Politeness.* Are they courteous on the phone and in person? Will they try to give you an appointment on the same day if you really need it? The same criteria that apply to good restaurants and other service organizations should certainly hold true at the beauty parlor. I think politeness is important; nobody has to tolerate rude, distracted personnel.

3. *Prices.* Don't be embarrassed to ask before you go. And be sure to find out exactly what the quoted price includes. Washing, blow drying, and conditioning are sometimes treated like expensive "a la" items whose cost is not included in the price of the cut.

4. *Tipping.* Many salons are evasive on this point, but you should persevere. You should know in advance whom you are expected to tip—does it include, in addition to the stylist, the persons who wash, blow dry?—and how much. Ask exactly how many people will be involved during your appointment and how much the standard tip is. Believe me, you'll be happy to know all this in advance.

5. *Services they perform.* Make sure they do what you want. Many establishments have a great reputation for cutting but do no coloring, or they may be acknowledged masters of the permanent and do, say, no frosting.

6. *Do they cut for men and women?* Some people find the presence of the opposite sex exciting; others don't care; others find it disconcerting. If you think you fall into the latter category, then ask ahead of time.

7. *Are the stylists men or women?* It's a fair question, for the same reasons stated above.

8. *Will you get the same person every time?* Maybe this is important to you; maybe it isn't. But you're certainly entitled to ask.

9. *Are appointments on time?* Some places run like clockwork; others are casual indeed about what you may have to do in the remainder of the afternoon.

10. *How long does the appointment take?* There are some people on a tight schedule who welcome the anonymity and efficiency of a fast-moving hairstyle salon. And there are others who savor an entire day of beautification liberally laced with gossip, chatting, magazine articles leisurely read. Make sure your expectations match the reality of the salon you call.

11. *When are they closed?* Sometimes it's the very day that would otherwise fit perfectly into your schedule. And sometimes they'll close down for summer vacation during the month you need the most beauty attention. Forewarned is forearmed.

12

Hair-Treatment Salons and Studios: Do They Really Work?

There's a category of establishments dedicated to the "improvement" of hair quality. Sometimes they're an adjunct to styling-and-cutting establishments, and sometimes they're in business all by themselves. The treatments they offer are so pleasant that I can't find it in my heart to be too negative. But the fact remains that many people go without fully understanding what these places can and cannot do.

I think it's a bad idea to decide spontaneously to undergo any "hair improvement" treatment, especially at the suggestion of an affable salon employee whom you may have just met. It's even a worse idea if this advice follows a "free" hair analysis. Better to pay for the analysis and get the straight story. Notwithstanding all protests to the contrary, anything "free" establishes a debt. At the very least it gives you a psychological predisposition to consider products or services of unknown value.

The typical treatment studio will sit you down in a private booth with a "trichologist," meaning one who studies and analyzes hair. Sometimes these analyses are impressive. They can include special infrared photos that supposedly point out deficiencies in certain hair elements ("Ms. X, your hair is clearly deficient in sulfur, so I'm recommending our special enrichment-conditioner program"). Some places have machines that test the hair's tensile strength to determine undue fragility, although you can do the same thing by stretching a single strand between your own two hands and noting whether it snaps with undue ease.

What's misleading here is the clinical pose. There is no test to become a "trichologist," nor are there any state or local licensing procedures. By the time you finish this book you'll be as much a trichologist as anybody.

What the treatment salons are selling is hope and a sense of pampered well-being, which is okay—unless a client thinks the establishment can cure a hair-loss problem. In more than nine cases out of ten, hair loss is strictly genetic and is a condition for which there is no hope. So it's suspicious indeed to see so many sufferers of thinning hair and baldness flocking to expensive hair-treatment salons.

If they really can't stop hair loss, then why doesn't the government shut them down? There is an artfully foggy concept that serves as the rationale for the studio hair-improvement industry. It's called *seborrheic dermatitis* (translation: "dandruff"). The salons and studios will all admit that there is nothing they can do for male pattern baldness. But they say they *can* improve seborrheic dermatitis. If you have that, they say, then you'll benefit from the treatments. And since everybody has some degree of dandruff, everybody is therefore a candidate for antiseborrhea techniques.

In rare cases hair loss actually does stem from seborrheic dermatitis. But if your scalp is that crusty, you should go to a doctor, not to a hair-treatment salon. Lately, many studios are acquiring a more medical look, and some even have doctors who consult on, say, hair transplants. But this shouldn't disguise their basic nonmedical nature. A hair analysis by a trichologist may or may not be as accurate as having a Gypsy read your palm. As for the published medical articles that are often shown to clients and that appear to buttress the treatment programs, just remember the old saying that the same statistics can prove any point of view. Doctors are besieged every day by mail solicitations to try various products on their patients. It's not uncommon to receive lucrative offers on a per-patient basis—fifty dollars apiece if you'll try such-and-such a product on two hundred patients. The thinking is that anything that's "doctor tested" is more marketable. So purveyors of products and services love to have themselves associated with a doctor's name. The point of all this is not that doctors are associating themselves with disreputable causes (they aren't recommending anything that will hurt anybody) but, rather, that it's a cinch to get a doctor's name in a published article. It's also easy to make something seem like an endorsement when it really isn't.

Having said this, I hasten to add that any studio will definitely be able to make dry, dandruffy hair much more manageable. You can spend a pampered afternoon having your hair conditioned and come out feeling like a million dollars. These places, as I've said, sell service, hope, and a sense of well-being. If you buy that without further illusions, I say go ahead and enjoy yourself.

MASSAGE

Massage is a big item at the salons, and everybody tells you how it promotes a healthy scalp. Well, a healthy scalp does *not* guarantee burgeoning tresses of healthy, luxurious hair. To be sure, certain scalp diseases (discussed in chapters 13 and 15) can affect the hair if they harm the follicles. But if you just have plain old garden-variety dandruff, it won't hurt your follicles, and a massage won't do much of anything for it, either. Genetics largely determine the quality of your hair; the condition of your scalp is important only if it's badly diseased.

Massage makes you feel relaxed and temporarily increases the blood supply on the scalp. However, the scalp is already so richly supplied that any temporary increase is superfluous. Certainly it won't do a thing for the way your hair is or isn't growing. Conclusion: Scalp massages are fun, but they have nothing to do with your hair.

ULTRAVIOLET LIGHTS

You'll hear them called sunlamps, blue lights, or my favorite from the standpoint of theatricality, cold quartz lamps. They all help seborrhea and seborrheic dermatitis, just as the sun does. What's more, they usually give off an encouragingly medicinal ozone smell, and you may even get a bit of a tan.

Sunlight and sunlamps are great for acne, seborrhea, and dandruff. The problem with salon treatments is that unless you go every day, you can't get the needed continuity. For it to be really effective, you have to sit in the sun or under a sunlamp *every day*. Missing days or doing it once a week or less renders ultraviolet-light treatments ineffective.

Since dandruff is the cornerstone of the hair-treatment studio, I refer you to Chapter 13, which contains many self-help suggestions for dandruff, including a sunlamp regimen. A serious course of home sunlamp treatments is much better than occasional exposure in a salon. Better yet is to sit in the sun daily.

SUPER DANDRUFF SHAMPOOS

Dandruff shampoos are actually more effective than sun-lamp treatments. Some salons suggest that their brands are particularly effective, but I don't believe this is true. In my opinion you can get the equivalent in any drugstore. The same companies supply both retail and professional markets with the same products. Only the labels are different.

CONDITIONING TREATMENTS

Unlike medical texts, cosmetology manuals waffle on the subject of what massages actually can do. But most operators accept everything in the beauty-school text and uncritically follow instructions on how to massage smoothly patrons who are undergoing conditioning treatments. Massages of the shoulders and vertebral column are intended to stimulate nerves and increase the blood supply to the scalp—despite the medical fact that increased blood supply does nothing. As for the stimulating massage, well, who doesn't enjoy that?

The operators who perform them are not cynical. They want to do a good job, and they probably believe the whole increased-blood-supply-and-stimulation story.

For dry-hair problems the massage manipulations are usually combined with the application of hot oils. The hair is washed, towel dried, and parted at the crown into approximately equal quadrants. The head is then anointed with heated oils or protein conditioners, put under a cap or a plastic steamer, then rinsed and shampooed.

This is practically identical with some of the do-it-yourself conditioning procedures described in Chapter 4. The only differences are the unnecessary massage and the substitution of salon steamer caps for the steaming hot towels you use at home. These conditioning treatments are a particularly good illustration of the basic weakness in the hair-improvement salons—namely, they can't do anything for you that you can't do yourself. There was a time, before the proliferation of cosmetic hair products, when you couldn't buy dandruff shampoos, body-building protein conditioners, and so forth. But that time is long gone.

If you have a dry scalp, plenty of money, and like to feel pampered, then by all means go to one of these places and have yourself a hot-oil deep-conditioning treatment. Just remember that you can do the same thing at home by yourself or with the help of a friend.

Wash and part the hair just as they do in the salons. The best conditioning oil is castor oil, which can be heated on your kitchen stove. Apply it hot to the hair, wrap the head in a steaming hot towel, wait ten to fifteen minutes, and shampoo with mild baby shampoo. This is just the sort of enjoyable self-improvement that two people can do with and to each other.

Unless your hair is very, very dry, it's doubtful you need hot-oil conditioning. There are plenty of conditioners and cream rinses that you can use in the shower together with your shampoo (there's a long list of these in Chapter 4). Dryness usually responds best to reducing the number of shampoos and brushing the hair regularly to distribute natural oils.

Part III
Medical Help for Your Hair—Common Problems and Cures

13

Diseases of the Hair and What the Doctor Can Do

Odds are there's nothing medically wrong with your hair. But an unlucky few do suffer from a dazzling variety of afflictions. Below are descriptions of the sixteen most common hair and scalp diseases, together with advice on what to do. Please note that this list does *not* include internal or systemic diseases whose symptoms affect the hair.

1. *Seborrheic dermatitis, or dandruff.* Dandruff and its stronger cousin psoriasis are both conditions that affect the skin's natural rate of cell turnover. Your skin grows from the inside out, meaning that new cells are manufactured in the lower layers of the epidermis. These cells gradually work their way to the surface and replace naturally shedding surface cells. The whole process is called skin-cell turnover.

People with dandruff have an unnaturally fast rate of cell turnover. This causes both redness and an accumulation of whitish flakes of shedding skin. It's so easy to treat dandruff that there's really no excuse to suffer its extreme unattractiveness. Drugstore shelves are full of effective nonprescription dandruff shampoos. Since the effectiveness of any medicine decreases the more you use it, I recommend that you buy two or three dandruff shampoos and use a different one each day. Here's a list of several good ones:

Zincon
Zetar
Sebulex
Vanseb T
Head 'n Shoulders
Enden
Selsun

Plenty of other dandruff products are equally good. All dandruff shampoos are strong, so you may notice your hair becoming dry and flyaway. That's why I recommend that you follow every dandruff shampoo with a cream rinse or conditioner.

Sunshine also helps dandruff. If you can, sit in the sun as much as possible, or get a sunlamp. Sunlamps should always be used with eye-protecting goggles, and the first exposure should not exceed five seconds. After that the exposure time should be increased five seconds every day until you hit a plateau of between two and three minutes, depending on skin tolerance. Use the lamp on the hair just as you would on the face. Keep it moving and don't let the rays shine on any one spot for uninterrupted periods.

Dandruff is also recurrent, so if you think you've whipped the problem, don't be disheartened if it comes back in a few months. Just treat it again with the shampoos and (if necessary) the sunlight. Only in very severe cases will a doctor's help be necessary.

There are times when seeming dandruff isn't dandruff at all. "Pseudodandruff" is a term that describes white dandruffy flecks in the hair that actually have a wholly different cause. Too much hair spray is a common culprit, as are flecks of hardened hair dressings. These, however, are easily removed with shampooing.

Another cause of pseudodandruff is an infestation of nits, which are little white mites that nest in the hair and set up housekeeping. Nits are not evidence of squalid living; regular shampoos just can't get them out of the hair. And mites can get into the hair during the most elegant of picnics; all you have to do is lie down on an unlucky patch of grass. The cure for this type of pseudodandruff is **Kwell,** a prescription product that comes in lotion and shampoo form. Kwell, incidentally, also removes lice.

2. *Psoriasis of the scalp.* Psoriasis is the most common skin disease after acne. It can affect any part of the body, and on the scalp its scaly and raised red crusts can be dangerous to your hair. Left untreated for too long a time, a bad case of psoriasis can permanently damage hair follicles and prevent future hair growth. But if you take care of the problem promptly, your hair and scalp both have a chance to return to normal.

Like dandruff, psoriasis often responds well to the sun or a sunlamp. The dandruff shampoos mentioned above are also helpful. Additionally, there's a good over-the-counter product called **P and S Solution,** which removes the crusts overnight. If the condition persists, you should definitely see a dermatologist.

3. *Fungus infections.* A fungus infection of the head is called *tinea capitis,* but fungi can attack hair on any part of the body. Minor epidemics are quite common. Any environment with kids, cats, and dogs can be a ready breeding ground. Once it starts, it spreads like wildfire. Sometimes entire classrooms are infected, teacher and all.

The fungus in cases of tinea capitis is ringworm. The little buggers invade the hair shaft and actually eat the keratin. Before you know it, the hair begins to crumble away, leaving white scaly bald patches on the scalp. People who let it persist risk scarring the scalp, sometimes damaging follicles to the point that they never grow hair again.

But treat it in time and you'll be fine. All fungi are treated the same, whether they are highly contagious, like ringworm, or not. The medicine of choice is an over-the-counter product called **Tinactin,** which comes in cream, liquid, and powder form. In severe cases your doctor can recommend a stronger prescription systemic medication, in pill form, called **Griseofulvin.**

4. *Impetigo of the scalp.* I think most mothers have had at least close brushes with impetigo, if not offspring with nasty cases. It's a highly contagious bacterial infection that regularly attacks young children at school or camp. It's not their youth but their dirty play environment which breeds the guilty bacteria.

In extreme cases impetigo of the scalp can have the same bad effects on follicles that we talked about above. It's very easy to treat, either with an OTC antibacterial shampoo called **Betadine** or with antibiotic pills prescribed by your doctor.

5. *Atopic eczema.* Like psoriasis, eczema can crop up on any part of the body. It's symptomized by varying degrees of redness, oozing, and weeping sores. When a condition like this hits the scalp, the hair thins and the follicles become vulnerable to possibly irreversible damage.

Eczema on the scalp responds well to sun and sunlamps. It also seems to be improved by an increase in humidity in the environment. If you live in the desert or spend your winters in centrally heated houses and offices, you should consider getting an electric humidifier. Setting out shallow tubs of water around the house, letting them evaporate naturally, and keeping houseplants also help humidify the environment. A mild, soothing paste like **Zinc Oxide** should be applied to the affected area, too—just a little dab will do. If things don't improve in a week, your doctor or dermatologist might try some sort of steroid treatment.

6. *Lichen planus*. The first half of the name is "lichen" because these flat-topped reddish or violet papules look like the lichens on a rock. Again, they can appear anywhere on the body, but on the scalp they can leave scars that pose a particular threat to the hair follicles. Lichen planus is a case of cell-turnover rate that is abnormally slow. The papules come in multiple groups and look pretty awful. You might think some sort of virus was at the root of this. Not so; the condition is believed to be related to stressful living. This is a disease that you should without delay see your doctor about. He'll treat it with prescription steroids, if possible, before your follicles suffer permanent damage.

7. *Alopecia areata*. This is a type of hair loss characterized by quarter-sized bald patches that appear amid otherwise healthy hair. The causes are rarely medical; rather, it is thought to be a mysterious reaction of the body to psychological stress.

Unlike cases of ringworm, the alopecia areata bald spots have no scaliness. Doctor-prescribed steroids—injected, swallowed, or applied directly to the affected area—sometimes help. Given the psychological element, the best cure is "tincture of time." Be patient, calm down, and your hair will usually grow back as mysteriously as it fell out.

8. *Growths*. The trouble with growths on the scalp lies in their capacity to obliterate the local hair follicles. Common ones include warts, skin cancers, and a very common and sometimes precancerous growth called a **sebaceous nevus.** Some people are born with one or more nevi, and others develop them later in life. They are usually yellowish, oily, and unwelcome. I advise you for the sake of your hair and overall appearance to have a doctor remove any growths promptly. Most of these procedures can be handled in the doctor's office.

9. *Keloids on the scalp.* Keloids are thick scars that occasionally occur spontaneously but are more often the result of some sort of trauma. On the head, these traumas can include anything from tick bites to bad burns to infected head wounds to badly ingrown hairs. Some people—especially black people—are particularly liable to keloids. When they occur on the scalp, keloids can take all the nourishment away from the follicles. And follicles starved for nourishment can't grow hair. Sometimes doctors can shrink keloids with steroid injections.

10. *Physical trauma.* Certain things that happen to your head can kill your follicles. Frostbite of the scalp is one example. X rays, especially the sort that were once used to treat ringworm infections, are another. Burning from fires or chemicals is a third. Overheated oils from hot-comb hair-straightening treatments so often cause hair loss that the condition has its own medical name—hot-comb alopecia.

As I've already mentioned, a common temporary physical cause of hair loss is *traction alopecia.* This term refers to pulling the hair out by unduly vigorous brushing and/or severely pulled-back hairstyles like ponytails or corn rows.

11. *Trichotillomania.* Perhaps you've watched somebody sitting listening or reading or talking, all the while languidly twisting a strand of hair. This nervous habit at its worst can turn into trichotillomania, or self-induced, personally plucked bald patches. By the way, it's not easy to convince people that their hair loss is caused entirely by the nervous twirling. They would much rather believe that they suffer from a physical ailment. The cure for trichotillomania—which, believe it or not, is exceedingly common—is relaxation and sometimes tranquilizers.

12. *Pseudopelade of Brocq.* The condition was first described by Brocq, but no one really understands it fully. The victims are mainly middle-aged men and women who begin to develop small bald patches. The skin is shiny and eventually develops follicle-destroying scars. Sometimes your doc-

tor can prescribe helpful steroids, but oftentimes there's not much that can be done.

13. *Lupus erythematosus.* Here's a familiar disease and I see it often indeed. Lupus can attack other parts of the body, but when it hits just the scalp or skin, it's called *discoid lupus.* The symptoms are early hair loss with no regrowth, and the diagnosis is easy to make for the following reason. When the doctor plucks a hair from a lupus sufferer, a small bit of skin surrounding the follicle opening also comes off with the hair. The plucked hair and its skin fragment look just like a carpet tack.

Interestingly, lupus is a photosensitive disease, so much of the treatment boils down to keeping out of the sun. In addition, your doctor may prescribe strong systemic steroids in pill form.

14. *Folliculitis.* Folliculitis is an inflammation of the hair follicles that can stem from a bacterial, viral, or almost any other type of infection. It happens frequently in unsanitary living environments. Antibacterial shampoos, like Betadine, and (sometimes) doctor-prescribed antibiotics can usually clear it up before it causes lasting damage.

15. *Majocchi granuloma.* This condition is an overreaction to a common yeast infection. You'll see it most often as little scaly patches on legs that have been shaved with dirty razors. The granuloma can destroy the hair follicle, but on legs this rarely matters. The unattractive patches routinely respond well to prescription antibiotics.

16. *Congenital atrichia.* Last and certainly least is the condition of being born totally without hair follicles in certain localized areas. This is surprisingly common and genetically caused. Usually there are just a few such spots, and they're easy to cover with adjoining hair. Persons with atrichia are ideal candidates for hair transplants, so if you have it and are really bothered, refer to Chapter 17 for details on the various hair-replacement techniques.

14

Nutrition and Your Hair

Perhaps the most important thing your follicles need to grow healthy hair is adequate calories. If your diet doesn't provide enough calories, your hair will show it. War refugees and anorexic Hollywood starlets occupy different extremes of the universe, but they both suffer from dull, brittle hair caused by calorie deprivation.

There's nothing wrong with going on a diet and losing weight. Too many people are too fat. But crash diets are out. I am a strong believer in counting calories, which is a little like learning a new but simple language. Please bear in mind that all the weird eat-all-you-want diets have follow-up maintenance periods that amount to nothing more than calorie counting.

Frankly, I think you should learn how to count calories, and count them all the time. If you're serious about maintaining an attractive weight, then the sooner you get yourself a little calorie book and start learning how much is in the food you eat, the better off you'll be. Most drugstores sell handy little pocket calorie counters. But for thorough listings buy a paperback copy of *The Brand Name Calorie Counter*, edited by Corinne Netzer and published by Dell, and/or *The Dictionary of Calories and Carbohydrates*, edited by Barbara Kraus and published by New American Library.

I believe the key to successful and permanent weight loss is patience. You can estimate the approximate number of calories it takes to maintain your current weight healthfully by multiplying that weight by fifteen. To lose weight, eat 20 percent fewer calories. Similarly, you can gain weight by eating 20 percent more. Cut down gradually, be patient, cut out breakfast maybe, get used to a little dullness, and don't cheat. Although simple calorie-counting diets are lacking in psychological crutches and razzmatazz, they will promote steady weight adjustment without damaging the hair.

Besides calories, hair follicles need sufficient amino acids, which are building blocks of proteins. Unfortunately, many fashionable health-food diets lack almost all of the essential amino acids. Without them follicles cannot fabricate hair. People with bad hair who go on strict vegetarian low-protein diets are making their hair worse. The sources of amino acids are exactly those high-protein foods they're cutting out—meat, milk, cheese, eggs.

Healthy hair production also requires adequate amounts of vitamin F. This is the name recently applied to essential fatty acids. From the standpoint of your hair, fat is a source of energy for both the metabolizing follicle and the oil glands that naturally condition and lubricate the hair. An average balanced diet gets sufficient vitamin F in the form of cooking oils and the fat in meat.

Certain essential minerals are intimately involved in good hair production. The most important is probably iron. It's also the mineral that women are most likely to lack. With birth-control pills, which interfere with the body's natural absorption of iron, and menstrual bleeding, women are always losing iron. The typical female has a lower blood count of iron than her male counterpart. Some studies have indicated that drugstore iron pills can help both hair and nails. So if your hair is dull and brittle, you might give iron pills a try, although nobody can guarantee their good effect.

An iron deficiency need not be very serious to cause poor-looking hair. You may well be subclinically deficient, meaning that your overall health is not threatened but that your bloodstream has an undesirably low iron content. Your doctor can give you two special tests to determine whether or not this is the case. One is called the serum iron test; the other is the total iron binding capacity test. These are simple and inexpensive blood tests that can determine whether or not you are deficient in iron. And they may be a good idea if you've tried everything else to cure breaking and falling hair. Where does the body get most of its iron? From red meat.

Sulfur is a ubiquitous element contained in almost everything, including amino acids and the hair itself. It's thought to maintain hair color. Most of the sulfur in our diet comes from leafy green vegetables. There's an old folk medicine called blackstrap molasses, laced with sulfur, which is benign and may be worth a try if you want to improve the quality of your hair color.

The human body contains a variety of trace elements, barely discernible amounts of minerals such as copper and zinc. Many people believe that a lack of these elements may hurt the hair. Selenium, a chemical element, is the focus of a current health-food craze which is based on a lack of it inducing cancer in laboratory rats.

There was a time in the not-too-distant past when the drinking water and food supplies naturally provided these trace elements. Not so anymore. With fluoridation, chemical fertilizers, and grain processing, the natural sources have been nearly eliminated. Most processed foods now have trace amounts of minerals added to them.

Besides calories, amino acids, fat, and minerals, the production of healthy hair also requires a full complement of vitamins. Fortunately, most normal, balanced diets will give you all the vitamins you need.

The B-complex vitamins are particularly important. These include, among others, thiamine (B-1), riboflavin (B-2), pyridoxine (B-6), and cyanocobalamin (B-12). The lack of any of them can cause things like dullness, scaling and redness of the scalp, dandruff, grayness, even baldness. We get our B-complex vitamins from green vegetables, pork, milk, yeast, unmilled wheat, liver, and beef.

Vitamin C is equally important. It maintains the capillaries that carry blood to your follicles. Without proper levels of vitamin C these capillaries will degenerate and hemorrhage. These *perifollicular hemorrhages,* as they are called, interrupt nutrition and disrupt the follicle's metabolic process.

The prime source of vitamin C is citrus fruits, and the relation between citrus fruits and bleeding was established by the English navy centuries ago. The bleeding gums and livid, hairless patches on the heads of seamen were eliminated when these sailors were required to eat limes—which is how the whole nation eventually came to be colloquially called limeys.

I mentioned earlier that follicles are extremely sensitive to hormones. Well, *androgen,* which is a male sex hormone—the equivalent female androgenic is called *progesterone*—is the ultimate follicle antagonist. Androgen inhibits follicle metabolism. In sufficient quantities it will shrink the follicle and put it permanently to sleep. This is what happens when people go bald. Their follicles aren't dead, but they've been anesthetized by high blood levels of androgen or—and this is important—substances *chemically similar* to androgen.

In some ways the body is like a black-and-white television set, which can't discriminate between shades of color. Follicles can mistakenly react to substances, such as certain vitamins, for example, whose chemical structure is similar to androgens. Vitamin E and some of the B-complex vitamins fall into this category. This is why it is thought certain vitamin pills may sometimes aggravate hair loss.

Everybody has a unique level of susceptibility to androgen. A given level of androgen or androgenic substances may have a big effect on one head but no effect at all on another. The liver is the organ that metabolizes androgen in both humans and animals. So if you eat liver, you can expect to ingest a substantial quantity of androgen. Most organ meats are androgenic, as are Rocky Mountain oysters and wheat germ. Most American beef is androgenic, too, because of doses of hormones typically fed to cattle during the fattening process.

It is pointless to attempt to list every single vitamin in the human diet. They all play small but important parts in hair growth. Recently there's been a craze for specially packaged vitamins for the hair. The manufacturers of hair vitamins point correctly to the relationships between vitamins and good hair. They cite cases of how certain vitamin and trace-mineral deficiencies cause hair loss or damage. These hair vitamins certainly can't hurt you. I think you should remember, however, that a normal, healthy body will automatically provide its hair follicles with every necessary vitamin and mineral. What you can do to safeguard this natural state is maintain homeostasis.

The human body is a terrific machine that is naturally homeostatic. This state is nothing more than a healthy status quo. No, the secret to beautiful hair does not lie in eating three pounds of anchovies every week, or in avoiding fried foods, or in any other exotic diet regimen. Just eat a normal, balanced diet, and your body will naturally produce all the necessary components for healthy hair growth.

Homeostasis is so much the natural order of things that it

takes an effort and/or an awful lot of bad luck to disrupt it. Hair that's brittle, dull, or falling out in clumps is often related to diabetes, pregnancy, overprocessing with strong chemical bleaches and dyes, and other factors. These things are the culprits far more often than diet. Of course, if you're already in ill health, your homeostasis is disrupted by definition. Your hair is therefore more vulnerable to diet deficiencies that might not otherwise have been serious enough to affect it.

Interestingly enough, pills are one of the most common causes of brittleness, dullness, and breakage of the hair. "Are you taking any medications?" is a question all doctors ask their patients. "No" is the usual answer. It continually amazes me that sane, thinking people don't consider things like aspirin, birth-control pills, and diet pills to be medication. Not only are these things medications, but they are prime causes of unnaturally bad hair as well. If a hair problem has brought you to the doctor, by all means tell him everything you are taking.

Hair and how it reacts to various medications will be fully treated in Chapter 15. For now I want to mention several of the most common drugs that can harm hair.

For some reason people often forget that these are medications.

The first is aspirin. Now, obviously you can take a couple of aspirin from time to time and they won't hurt your hair. There are people, however, who are practically addicted to aspirin. They erroneously believe it to be so bland as to be harmless. Well, if you take two aspirin every single night before you go to bed, there is a chance that your hair will become dull and start to fall out.

Birth-control pills have many unpredictable effects on the hair. Taking them may cause hair to fall out. And when taking them doesn't, stopping them may. Hair follicles are highly sensitive to hormones, and birth-control pills are practically pure hormone. Fortunately, you can easily change to a different pill if your doctor tells you that your present type is harming your hair.

Many other medications are the unsuspected cause of hair problems. Diet pills and amphetamines can make hair fall out. Cortisone, used to treat allergic reactions and arthritis, can cause hair simultaneously to grow on the face and fall from the scalp. Anticoagulants, which thin the blood, hormone injections to induce postpregnancy menstruation, and HCG, a drug injected for weight loss, can all cause problem hair loss.

The key concept in this chapter is that hair nutrition comes from within. Hair follicles are located deep in the dermis layer of the skin. This layer is located well below the surface and is protected from the environment by many layers of epidermal cells. It's your bloodstream that provides a balanced diet of vitamins, proteins, and hormones to your follicles. I hear stories of people rubbing everything from crude oil to crushed avocados on the head to improve or to grow hair. Given the physical location of hair follicles and the nature of the hair growth that occurs within them, it is impossible to "feed" them by rubbing anything on the scalp. Protein and oils will coat the hair and make it look temporarily better. Hormone injections can stimulate dormant follicles, but they may be carcinogenic. There is no externally applied substance that can safely affect either the rate of hair growth or the quality of the hair produced.

The hair follicle is one of the body's most rapidly metabolizing organs. This means that it goes about its business of digesting nutrients and producing hair at an extremely fast rate. It's also true that changes—either for the better or for the worse—take a long while to show up in the hair. There is no paradox here. Hair growth is very slow and it can take weeks or even months for changed hair to grow out and become noticeable.

Your chances of being in homeostasis right now are exceedingly good, and your diet is probably perfectly satisfactory. There *is* no diet especially for the hair. Eat whatever you want, just as long as your diet is balanced.

Part IV
Why Hair Falls Out—and What You Can Do About It

15

The Medical Causes of Hair Loss

It's normal to lose from 100 to 200 hairs daily as part of the hair's normal growth-and-shed cycle. It's also common—although hardly normal—to tease, tangle, bleach, and otherwise overprocess the hair to the point where it breaks off. But in addition to natural cycles and physical abuse, there are a number of medical conditions that deplete the hair. What follows is a discussion of the seven most important such conditions.

1. *Male pattern baldness.* Baldness occurs in women, too. Male pattern baldness is more common in men, but the factors that cause it are all present in women. Your genetic heritage is the foremost cause, specifically the inherited hair-follicle sensitivities to certain hormones. Your follicles' worst enemy is the male sex hormone androgen. Unopposed, androgen will counter follicle metabolism and essentially put the follicle permanently to sleep. The female sex hormone estrogen naturally counteracts androgen. However, in addition to estrogen, the female ovaries and adrenals produce their own androgenlike hormone called progesterone.

Normal men usually lose their hair because their follicles

cannot tolerate the levels of androgen in their bloodstreams. The situation is slightly different in women. For them advancing years are usually reflected in decreased levels of estrogen. When this happens, the woman's androgenlike progesterone finds itself unopposed. Depending on the sensitivity of the hair follicles—and here's where inherited strengths are important—the unopposed androgenic progesterone levels can cause the same sort of hair loss frequently seen in men.

Genetic baldness follows a typical pattern—the hair thins at the crown while the hairline simultaneously recedes on the temples. There are individual variations on this general pattern, depending on the inherited sensitivities of the follicles on different parts of the scalp. But current medical thought ascribes all the aging-balding patterns to the unopposed effect of either androgen itself or other androgenic hormones. There's really nothing a man can do to reverse this natural process. Women, however, can avail themselves of estrogen therapy, an admittedly controversial subject, described at the end of this chapter.

2. *Poor diet.* Hair follicles need calories, fats, amino acids, minerals, and vitamins to grow hair. Deny the body these needed nutrients and your hair will become dull and brittle— or it might stop growing altogether. "Cachectic" (pronounced ka-*kek*-tik) is a wonderful word in the medical vocabulary that describes diets so intensely nonnutritive that they can bring the dieter to the verge of starvation. Suffice it to say that the frantically fashion-conscious often subsist on cachectic diets. The damage they cause to the hair is reversible by substitution of a balanced diet.

3. *Certain medications.* Many medications are either androgenic or make the hair fall out for other reasons. Baldness is uncommon enough among women that at the first sign of substantial hair loss you should ask yourself what pills or medicines you're taking. Here are some common culprits.

Aspirin (rare)
Anticoagulants of the blood (two common examples are
    coumadin and heparin)
Dilantin (used most frequently for epileptic seizures)
Amphetamines
Certain anticancer drugs (used in chemotherapy)
Thyroid pills
Birth-control pills (these have an eccentric effect; some
    women never have any problems, whereas others have
    nothing but; progesterone pills have been associated
    with hair loss in some women)
Cortisone (and all steroids used to treat arthritis, as well as
    various aches and inflammations)
Boric acid (much overused because it seems so benign;
    contained in eyewashes, soothing ointments for burns
    and cuts, and many mouthwashes)

Ingesting any of these substances certainly does not automatically mean that your hair will fall out. The effect
depends on the vulnerabilities of your own follicles.

4. *Major shocks or changes.* Having a baby is a major
bodily shock; so are being hit by a bus, ending a long-term
nonstop course of birth-control pills, and losing a parent.
Major traumas that lead to large-scale *telogen effluvium* can
be either physical or psychological. Telogen effluvium, once
again, is the normal hair fallout that occurs during the
telogen phase of the growth-and-shed cycle. Normally only a
small proportion of follicles are in the phase at any given
time. But major traumas can terminate the anagen growth
phase in an abnormally large number of follicles. As these
follicles shrink, the hair begins to shed. In extreme cases
people can become completely bald and the hair can grow
back white. This is the origin of the description of a person's
hair turning white with fright. Actually, the hair all fell out,
then grew back white.

Big shocks usually stop far short of causing complete baldness. And the follicles will normally start to resume hair growth within two to three months. Even when the new hair is white, it will regain its natural coloration with the passage of time. The effluvium itself is a positive sign. It means the telogen phase has ended, and new anagen hair is pushing the old telogen shafts out of the follicle to make way for new growth.

5. *Alopecia areata.* As many as ten people a day come to my office with this condition. Some doctors think it's related to stress; others think it's connected to thyroid disease or deficiencies of vitamin B-12; still others put forth the theory that this particular type of hair loss is caused by a temporary allergy to one's own hair. As the variety of opinion indicates, the real causes are as mysterious as the condition is common.

Alopecia areata looks like quarter-sized bald patches which appear amid otherwise healthy hair. They are clearly demarcated, and sufferers usually get more than one at a time. Fortunately, they usually go away by themselves, although the first new hair that appears will more likely than not be white. This, too, is temporary. As the hair continues to grow, normal color reappears on the new growth.

Doctors sometimes prescribe mild anti-inflammatory creams or cortisone injections or steroid pills to counter the theoretical allergic reaction. But it's hard to tell whether or not these measures work, since the condition can usually be expected to go away by itself.

6. *Iron-deficiency anemia.* Iron is a particularly important participant in the chemical processes that take place in rapidly metabolizing organs. Since hair follicles are among the body's fastest metabolizers, it therefore follows that iron deficiency should seriously affect, possibly even stop, follicle metabolism. This theory hasn't been completely proved, but, like many things in medicine, it's an informed guess. The

body needs only a trace or a dash of so many things—iron, selenium, zinc, for example—but these elements are nonetheless considered critical to good health.

It's actually common for otherwise healthy women to have a subclinical iron deficiency, which is distinct from the radical deficiencies found in people whose whole lives are spent on the verge of starvation. Many women eat quite well, but with food preferences and regular menstruation they can still be subclinically deficient. Which is to say, they lack iron but not very much.

Two simple blood tests can easily determine whether a gradually growing hair-loss problem is related to iron deficiency or not. The first is called the serum iron test, and it measures the total amount of iron contained in the bloodstream. The second is the serum total iron-binding capacity test, which shows the ratio of the amount of iron in the blood to the blood's total capacity to hold iron. A normal ratio is about 1 to 4. A really iron-deficient ratio would be 1 to 7. If you fall somewhere in between and your hair is looking poor and falling out, you might well benefit from iron therapy.

This therapy consists of taking little green pills called ferrous gluconate, or iron pills. They are cheap, require no prescription, and have mild side effects. About the most upsetting of these seem to be the black stools that result from the typical two-pills-per-day treatment. Some people also experience an increase in appetite, general nausea, sometimes constipation. But usually the black stool is the sole side effect. Read the instructions on the label.

Although iron pills are available without prescription, it doesn't make much sense to take them for hair loss unless you've undergone the tests above. The tests are well known and cost about $20 for both, in addition to the doctor's normal fee.

7. *Acute or chronic disease.* Anytime you're seriously sick you can expect some degree of hair loss. Here are some examples of the types and degree of sickness necessary.

Diabetic coma
A big car crash or any other major accident
A major infection (such as pneumonia or flu)
Acute depression or schizophrenia
Chronic bleeding ulcers (these can lead to iron deficiency; interestingly, a doctor can reconstruct the incidence of bleeding attacks by examining the hair shaft for beads, since the hair stops growing during a bleeding attack and leaves a bead when it resumes)
Liver disease (the liver metabolizes androgens; damage like that sustained by years of heavy drinking can allow unopposed androgens to close down the hair follicles; this is the only medical cause of hair loss that looks just like male pattern baldness)
Cachexia (starvation)
TB
Colitis (this is an inflammation of the large bowels that denies nutrient absorption into the bloodstream)
Malignancy (cancerous tumors siphon off nutrients in the blood and deny the hair follicles food)
Hypo/hyperthyroid disease (diffuse hair loss is related to conditions of either too much or too little thyroid in the system)
Diabetes (when the body can't properly metabolize carbohydrates, blood-sugar levels can go on wild swings that interfere with hair nutrition)

A HAIR-LOSS CHECKLIST

If you think you're losing your hair for a medical reason, read this checklist before you do anything.

1. *Don't panic.* The normal daily loss rate of 100 to 200 hairs can look like more than it is. Especially if you shampoo every three days, then 300 to 600 hairs in the shower drain may make you frightened for no reason. Be calm and don't let hairs in the drain convince you that your luxurious hair is on the verge of extinction.

2. *Review the last three months.* On the other hand, there may really be medical causes or new health developments that are affecting your hair. Ask yourself if you've started taking any new medications, if you've been sick or under undue stress, if you've changed your eating habits. If you suspect some medication, your doctor may be able to prescribe an effective substitute that won't harm the hair.

3. *See a doctor.* He can give you tests for iron deficiency, thyroid levels, blood sugar, and hormone levels. He's the last resort when everything else leaves you baffled. Even if you live in a remote locale without lab facilities, your doctor can still give you the tests. The Bioscience Lab in California, for example, does certain blood-analysis tests for doctors as far away as New York.

ESTROGEN THERAPY

If all the tests are negative, then you're probably on the genetically determined path to partial or total baldness. There's no hope for men, at least at present, but women can always investigate estrogen therapy.

There are two approaches to the therapy, and they're

employed either independently or jointly. The first involves the topical application of an estrogen lotion called **Premarin**. You rub the Premarin into the scalp, following the doctor's directions, and then wait and see. There's very little systemic absorption with Premarin lotion, but there might be enough to counter the levels of androgenic hormones in the hair follicles. Then again, there might not be.

Alternately, you can either begin a course of estrogen-type birth-control pills or take pure-estrogen Premarin pills. This gets the estrogen into the blood but carries significantly higher risk of undesirable side effects.

The effects and side effects of estrogen are not easy to predict. If it stops hair loss at all, it will do so only by means of opposing an otherwise unchecked androgen effect. Sometimes this works only to the point of stopping a high rate of hair loss; other times the estrogen therapy actually seems to promote new hair growth; and other times the therapy can actually make the hair fall out.

Men can't take estrogen because it encourages a host of secondary female sex characteristics. However, in women and especially menopausal and postmenopausal women these characteristics are desirable. Estrogen can preserve and promote a wonderful, sexy glow on skin, hair, and breasts. It even seems to ease the psychological stress associated with menopause.

On the other hand, hormones are tricky substances, and introducing them into the bloodstream is not without risk. Cancer, blood clots, increased veins on the face, and tumors in the uterus are only a few of the bizarre things that can happen. This is not to say that these awful things definitely accompany all estrogen therapy. And the risk is apparently acceptable enough to the many thousands of women who undergo the therapy. As for the future, who knows? Scientific miracles regularly happen. It may not be long before estrogen risks are dramatically reduced or a safer androgen antagonist is developed.

16

Calm Down and Grow Hair

A certain amount of stress is a natural part of life until it activates what's called the "fight or flight" mechanism—a throwback to when we lived in the bushes and frightening things prowled around us. Fight or flight is a specific reaction pattern: Logic declines; the heart pumps at a faster rate; blood vessels close to the skin constrict; the hair stands on end; perhaps most importantly, the adrenal glands pump the system full of a powerful hormone called adrenaline.

Adrenaline is the remarkable emergency hormone that's credited with giving frail mothers the strength to lift fallen cars off teenage-son mechanics, and aged refugees the endurance to sprint across borders. But besides adrenaline, your adrenals produce androgenic sex hormones, and herein lies the hair problem. A current hypothesis is that these androgenic hormones can anesthetize your follicles and make your hair fall out. The adrenal glands secrete nonspecifically, which means that whenever they are stimulated, they'll let loose with a whole package of hormones. This package includes not only adrenaline but also the sometimes unneeded and unwanted androgens.

To make things worse, your adrenals can start pumping

even without the presence of muggers, wild animals, or sinister secret police. Feedback from the brain constantly influences adrenal secretion. If your brain is suffering from stressful delusions or neurotic convictions, your body will show it. The best illustration of this is pseudopregnancy, in which a woman is so convinced she's pregnant that she will actually miss her period, become heavier, and manifest all sorts of other pregnancy symptoms.

In my office, nine out of every ten women complaining of diffuse hair loss turn out to be under undue emotional tension. We're not talking about male pattern baldness here; this diffuse hair loss is not limited to specific areas and is not a matter of genetics.

At first a chronic accumulation of stress can be as un-noticeable as gradual stress-related hair loss. About 10 percent of an average head's 100,000 hairs must fall out before the condition becomes apparent. Because hair grows slowly, one to three months can pass between a succession of stressful events and the first sign of resulting hair loss. And these stressful events don't have to be earthshaking. Besides divorce and trauma are marriage, having kids, starting a new business, moving to a new house. Minor things can add up, too: business being bad or business being good, minor sex problems, hassles with neighbors.

Psychological stress can also lead to physically stressful habits such as drinking too much or existing on a non-nutritious diet. There can be a double-whammy effect, wherein your stress-stimulated adrenals saturate your blood-stream with follicle-deadening androgen-like compounds while your diet denies those same follicles the nutrients necessary to grow good hair. On top of this, many people tend to become a little neurotic at the first sign of hair loss. Automatically they start overtreating, overwashing, overteas-ing, overbrushing, and overdoing just about everything in a misguided effort to make things better.

My point here is not that inducing a Madonna-like calm will improve everybody's hair. But it's usually true that a chronically stressful life is the cause of diffuse hair loss. Recognizing this connection is the first step toward improving it.

CALMING DOWN

Telling people to calm down is a little like urging them to be free (easy to say and hard to do). But if your hair is falling out in fistfuls and you spend every waking hour in agonizing anxiety, then clearly you should do something. Your hair is really secondary to your own long-range mental health. It's one of the body's signals that unsupportable levels of stress have been reached. You might be able to keep the lid on things for the short run, but eventually something more serious than your hair is going to give.

Calming down often means major change. Sometimes it's your environment or your job or your psychotherapist—or even your spouse. Just taking a first step can give you a needed decompression, whether or not you finish what you start. Try anything reasonable—it's making a move that counts.

Usually the prescription is much less drastic. For example, exercise is a great stress reducer, which may account for the recent phenomenal growth in the popularity of participation sports. Whether you play tennis or squash, chop wood or bowl, jog every morning or ski in the Rockies, the physical outlet is bound to be tension reducing. Also relaxing are hobbies, which can include everything from playing the piano to collecting stamps to knitting and crocheting.

If you feel you might be suffering stress-related hair loss to a really serious degree, then go to a doctor. For one thing, he can give you tests which will establish whether or not there's another medical reason for hair loss. And he can also prescribe the most American of cures, a pill. Valium, for example, is not only safe, it's a widely used and effective calmative.

In some cases the only effective approach is psychiatry or psychotherapy. This assumes that there's a lot more troubling you than just simple stress and that your falling hair is a symptom of something bigger. Some people still cling to archaic prejudices against psychological help. I'm sure everyone's heard someone disdainfully proclaim that certain things simply have to be solved on one's own. There is an underlying assumption here that human problems are something to be ashamed of. Often the people who express these sentiments are those most ashamed of themselves.

If that's not discouraging enough, the task of finding psychological help or its high cost can be just as frustrating. In that case you may want to consider the psychiatric walkin clinics found in most big hospitals. Going to one of these places does *not* mean you're crazy. Quite the contrary. It shows you have sense enough to seek help when life is weighing you down. The mere act of walking in the door on your own makes you an ideal candidate for free hospital psychiatry, either singly or in a group. Hospital psychiatric staffs figure that psychological approaches work best on people with insight. If you have enough insight to feel you need help, that's often enough to get you into a program. Many of these programs are not only enlightening but even— believe it or not—fun. In lieu of this, maybe you have a friend in therapy who is enthusiastic about his or her therapist and can't wait to recommend this person.

Even when you do successfully calm down, don't expect your hair to improve or regrow overnight. It took months to show damage in the first place, and it'll take months to improve. Most of it will probably have to fall out before healthy new growth becomes obvious.

A RECAPITULATION OF HAIR DISEASES WHICH MAY BE RELATED SPECIFICALLY TO STRESS

1. *Alopecia areata.* In this condition the hair falls out from either stress or fright. The mechanism is not fully understood, but it's thought that the body somehow develops a temporary allergy to its own hair. The hair loss can occur in several well-demarcated patches amid otherwise healthy hair or, in extreme cases, the whole head can go bald. The loss is temporary and new hair eventually grows back. Surprisingly, the new hair is usually white. But after a while the normal color returns. Incidentally, it is impossible to get diffuse grayness from stress or worry. Grayness, like male pattern baldness, is determined genetically and there's nothing you can do to prevent it.

2. *Trichotillomania.* The hallmark of this stressful condition is constant unconscious twirling and tugging of the hair, resulting in little bald patches. This is a hard one to treat, mostly because it's obviously a symptom of more serious psychological problems. Some doctors have tried suturing, or stitching, bandages onto the affected area. Frankly, I think this is risky—remove this symptom, and who knows what the next one will be? Sometimes trichotillomania sufferers must undergo years of psychotherapy; sometimes the disease just goes away by itself.

3. *Dandruff and psoriasis.* These are both conditions of a too-rapid cell-turnover rate, and stress can make them worse. Mild or normal cases won't hurt your follicles, but extreme cases made worse by relentless chronic accumulated stress can sometimes obliterate the follicles and/or leave scars that prevent future hair growth.

4. *Lichen planus.* These reddish-purplish papules get their name because they resemble lichens on a rock. The disease is a case of skin cells reproducing too slowly, and it's com-

monly connected with stress. In fact, a death in the family is the most common cause of a case of lichen planus. The papules can appear anywhere on the body, but on the scalp they can leave scars that obliterate the follicles.

5. *Increased capillary fragility.* Fragile capillaries are more liable to break before they deliver nutrient-rich blood to the hair follicles. Stress is again connected to a tendency toward capillary fragility. If significant numbers of your capillaries are breaking, you can literally starve your follicles. Result: no hair growth.

17

Hair Replacement

Baldness in both sexes is a matter of what's called *end-organ sensitivity*. The end organ is the hair follicle, and its genetically determined sensitivity to androgenic sex hormones is what's in question. Some follicles are supposedly more sensitive to androgen than others. These more sensitive follicles are thought to stop growing hair when blood levels of androgenic hormones rise above their sensitivity threshold. But at the same time, other follicles elsewhere on the head will usually be able to tolerate the higher androgen levels and continue to grow hair.

The androgen effect is the same in men and women. The only difference is that of degree. Without being killed, the hair follicles shrivel and become dormant. As long as a woman's system is producing female estrogenic hormones in sufficient quantities, she will be able to combat the androgen effect. But as the woman's body ages, and especially after menopause, her natural levels of estrogen begin to fall. There is a point, unique for every woman, beyond which her estrogen and estrogenic hormones can no longer combat her androgenic hormones. If and when she ever reaches that point, some of her follicles may stop producing hair, depending, of course, on their individual sensitivities to androgen.

If baldness or substantial thinning is going to happen, it's rare to see it before the beginning of the fourth decade of life. Usually it comes later than that. In Chapter 15 we talked about estrogen therapy, which many women swear by. But, although estrogen certainly inhibits androgen in the bloodstream, it also carries certain dangers—notably cancer. This is why many women won't take estrogen for the hair any more than they'd take it in birth-control pills.

Fortunately, in lieu of stoic acceptance of hairlessness or a possibly dangerous course of estrogen therapy, there are several very good alternatives.

HAIR TRANSPLANTS

Women are often much better candidates for hair transplants than men. This is ironic, since many people think a transplant is a procedure exclusively for males. Well, it isn't, not only because women are rarely as bald as men but also because female heads tend to have a more luxurious hair growth on the sides, where the transplant plugs are taken from.

How do you discover whether or not you are a good candidate for a hair transplant? This is a question you must take to a transplant expert. Generally speaking, transplants are not good for diffuse thinning all over the head. They're good for particularly thin or bare spots, and the more clearly demarcated, the better. Any licensed doctor, including but not limited to dermatologists and plastic surgeons, can perform a hair transplant. But if there was ever a cosmetic procedure whose good effect depended on experience, it's a hair transplant. The more transplants a doctor does, the better at it he or she will become. This sort of specialization is common in medicine, and in this case I feel I should stress its value. By the way, a doctor who does one transplant a week is *not* doing a lot of them.

Usually another doctor is the best person to ask for a recommendation. Just as your dentist will send you to someone else for root-canal work, so your regular doctor is best qualified to direct you to a transplant expert. I suppose there are some doctors who won't let a patient go to anybody else. But I think you can generally assume that if someone else is more experienced, an ethical doctor will recommend that person.

The transplant procedure itself does not require hospitalization; it is uncomfortable but not overly painful. The area that the plugs are to be taken from is anesthetized with simple novocaine injections. Usually this area is in the back of the head, in the midst of the thickest hair growth. The plugs are removed with an instrument called a hair-transplant punch, which makes round plugs, each of which measures about three and a half millimeters in diameter and contains eight to ten follicles. After they're removed from the scalp, the plugs are cleaned and trimmed of excess fat, then the doctor uses the same punch to prepare receiving holes in the transplant site. The cleaned plugs are fitted into the identically sized holes, which are spaced at least three and a half millimeters from one another. If they were any closer, the scalp's blood supply would be too disrupted for the transplanted plugs to heal properly.

The trauma of the transplant knocks the follicles in the transplanted plugs into the telogen phase. Shortly after, the transplanted hairs all fall out. But within three months, the scalp will have healed, the follicles will have embarked on a new anagen growth phase, and you can expect to see noticeable hair growth where there was formerly none. Some doctors reinsert the hairless plugs into the holes left by the transplanted ones; others don't. It doesn't matter if the holes are filled or not, since the scar tissue that forms over them will eventually be completely absorbed by the body. As it's absorbed, the surrounding tissues will be pulled together, leaving only a hairline scar where the transplanted plug was taken.

It's not possible to finish a transplant job in one sitting. Some doctors do only twenty-five plugs at a time, but even if you get a transplant specialist who does three or four times that number, you'll have to count on coming back. Average transplants involve anywhere from one hundred to five hundred plugs or more, and it's typical to come back three or four times over a period of years.

The cost is high—anywhere from $7.50 to $20 *per plug*. But the final effects typically are terrific-looking and durable. After all, it is your own hair. Since the procedure is not major, you usually won't even require a bandage after it's over. What's even better, federal income-tax laws have been recently changed to make the cost of cosmetic procedures— such as face lifts and hair transplants—tax deductible. This alone can make the whole project much more feasible.

I put great store in the traditional doctor-patient relationship. This is why I think you should personally search out a transplant specialist, perhaps through your doctor's recommendation. There are places, however, that hire doctors to perform transplants in quasi-medical salons or centers. The practitioners are certainly qualified, but these places sometimes lack a personal touch that I think is important.

HAIR IMPLANTS

In this procedure wefts, or swatches, of hair, sometimes your own, are attached to the scalp by means of Teflon-covered sutures. The implant procedure has several advantages over a transplant: 1) the job can be done considerably faster, usually in one visit; 2) it's much more comfortable; 3) when the job's completed, you've got immediate satisfaction. There's no prolonged wait for transplanted plugs to heal and new hair to grow. As soon as the doctor is finished with the implant, you'll get the finished effect.

On the other hand, there are drawbacks. There is a chance—albeit a minimal one—that you'll have a *foreign-body reaction* to the sutures. In this case you might experience considerable irritation, inflammation, and discomfort that won't be relieved until the sutures are removed. It's also hard to keep implanted hair tucked under a suture clean. More dirt and oil tend to collect on the scalp and resist shampooing, and this can sometimes lead to unpleasant odors.

Once again, implants are not recommended for diffuse hair loss on the entire head. They look best when used in certain clearly demarcated sparse or bald areas. They also cost almost as much as transplants, even though it seems as though they should cost less.

I think the safest way to find a doctor who has lots of experience in implants is to ask your own family physician for a recommendation. There are pseudo-medical hair establishments around that offer this service, but I would always ask my own doctor first. And it may well be that he will recommend the same local hair establishment that advertises in the newspapers and on TV.

HAIR WEAVING

Hair weaving is a process of tying new hair to old hair that's still rooted in your scalp. Sometimes a lattice is tied down first and the replacement hairs are threaded through it. And sometimes the weave is anchored completely on your own hair.

The big advantages to this process are its complete painlessness and its nonmedical nature. The initial cost is only a fraction of that of a transplant or implant; however, the low initial cost is just the first step. Once you get a hair weave, you've obligated yourself to continual maintenance costs, since every few weeks your weave must be reknotted closer to the scalp to allow for natural hair growth.

Where can you find out more about hair weaving? Ask your beauty parlor, look in the Yellow Pages, or ask your doctor to recommend a place.

WIGS

The tremendous technological advances of the last twenty-five years—mostly in the development of inexpensive synthetics—have revolutionized the wig industry. Annual wig sales passed the half-billion-dollar mark at the beginning of the 1970s, and the growth trend still continues.

As the prices have come down the convenience has apparently become irresistible. For openers, a good wig is almost undetectable, especially when it is artfully melded with the natural hair. Wigs can also eliminate time-consuming visits to a hair stylist. Even though you do have to send your wig to a beauty parlor periodically, at least you don't have to sit around and wait for it. A good wig can also give you a new look in moments, which is ideal for people who lead fast-paced lives.

To be officially considered a wig, a hairpiece must cover 80–100 percent of the head. Less than 80 percent coverage makes it a toupee, a term that is never used in connection with women. Wigs—as we'll call them for the sake of convenience—come in many shapes besides the 80–100 percent variety. There are, for example, postiches, which are small, round-based ornamental pieces made from angora or yak hair. Then there are wiglets, also small and usually curly, that embellish cocktail-party hairstyles. There are also chignons, long tresses piled in curls at the back of the head to add height and volume; falls, glamorizing hair that is added to your own hair and usually anchored on the crown of the head; mini-falls, and cascades, a mini-mini-fall that's four to eight inches in length.

All wigs are divided into two categories: human hair and synthetic. Human-hair wigs cost more and are considered superior in appearance and manageability. Naturally, not all human hair is the same. Some wigs are made with European hair, which is the easiest to style and the most expensive; others are made with either Oriental or Indian hair, which is coarser, a bit harder to manage, and has a tendency to curl. The location of the wig factory does not mean that's where the hair came from. It is not uncommon for a wig advertised as "imported from France" to be made of inexpensive human hair from South Korea. And, by the same token, some excellent-quality European-hair wigs are, for reasons of cost, manufactured outside Europe.

Synthetic wigs are much cheaper, but they'll never really look as good as the real thing. The trouble with artificial hair is its tendency to oxidize. Even human hair oxidizes and the colors dull, but rarely to a noticeable degree. By the way, this is just as much a problem with synthetic implants and hair weaves. When a wig is brand new it can be hard to tell a synthetic from the real thing. One sure test is to pluck a single strand and hold it over a lighted match. The synthetic fiber will melt and form a bead; a human hair will quickly frazzle and leave an unpleasant sulfurous odor. In most places you probably won't have to—let alone be able to—try this test. Still, it's useful to know of if you're engaged in heavy comparative shopping for a high-priced hairpiece.

Besides type of hair, wigs are also categorized by the way in which they are tied. Hand-tied wigs are more expensive and supposedly easier to manage. Machine-tied wigs are cheaper, and they may well be just as easy to manage.

The life-span of a wig varies according to quality and usage, but most of them become exhausted within one to three years. During the active life-span of human-hair wigs you must care for them sometimes just as assiduously as you care for your own hair. They need to be washed, set, sometimes colored, always by beauty-parlor professionals, and occasionally even cut by stylists. Many women buy quality hairpieces through their hairdresser, who then custom cuts the piece specifically for the customer. Since top-of-the-line prices for human-hair wigs are frequently way over $1,000, you won't want to be stingy on maintenance costs. It's a serious investment.

Wig cleanings are usually needed after eight to ten wearings. Mostly it's a function of the oiliness of your own scalp and the cleanliness of your environment, which includes things like air pollution. Beauty parlors use special cleaning fluids for human-hair wigs, and even though you can get these fluids for home use, I don't think it's worth the risk. The wrong cleaner can separate the hair from the base, and then there are conditioning and setting to consider. Unless you're really a pro, you're endangering your original investment by trying to do these things yourself.

Synthetic wigs are another story. These you can wash at home in lukewarm water and hang to dry on the bathroom doorknob. Some manufacturers even tell you to go ahead and throw them into the washing machine. As for price, you might find a small synthetic wiglet that's just what you want for under $20, although better grades and larger sizes cost substantially more.

All wigs should be kept on blocks when not in use. These blocks are shaped like bald human heads and they're usually made of white plastic. You really need two wigs, so you'll have a spare when the other is at the beauty parlor. Unused wigs should be draped with a scarf to ward off dust and stored in a loose-topped box or on a closet shelf to protect them from sun fading. Rain, incidentally, won't permanently damage a wig, but it will necessitate resetting any curls, because wig styles are water set to avoid damage from permanent-wave chemicals.

Probably the biggest drawback to a wig is discomfort. Some people can't stand the heat, others get headaches. This is an important consideration, which may well make you decide on another form of hair replacement.

Part V
What You Can Learn from Your Hair

18

The Do-It-Yourself Home Hair Analysis

The following two-part test is designed to be just like a visit to the doctor. Part I is equivalent to a typical preliminary office interview, in which the doctor learns your medical history and the circumstances surrounding your complaint. Part II corresponds to the traditional physical examination which follows the interview. But instead of talking to a doctor, I want you to conduct your own analysis, either by yourself or, particularly in Part II, with the help of a friend. A final note: I think you'll get more benefit from the simple, basic test questions in Part I if you answer them all *before* reading the Answer Notes that follow.

Part I. Medical History

SECTION 1. QUESTIONS

1. How old are you?
2. What color are your eyes?

3. What is your race?
4. What is the quality of your parents' hair?
5. How much do you brush your hair?
6. How many hairs do you lose per day?
7. Is your hair normal, oily, or dry?
8. How often do you shampoo?
.9. Do you think your hair grows rapidly, slowly, or at a normal rate?
10. How long is your hair?
11. What is the climate where you live?
12. What is the physical environment like where you work?
13. Are you active in sports?
14. Are you often in a nervous state?
15. What is the state of your health?
16. Are you taking any medications?
17. How would you describe your diet?
18. Are you pregnant or have you just had a baby?
19. Are your menstrual periods regular?
20. Do you blow dry your hair?
21. Do you color your hair?
22. How much time do you spend on your hair?

SECTION 2. ANSWER NOTES

1. *How old are you?* Hair naturally changes with age. For instance, much hormonally induced hair loss often occurs during adolescence and menopause. Adolescent hair loss is usually temporary; menopausal hair loss can be permanent, but the victims may be prime candidates for hair-restoring estrogen therapy. As the postmenopausal years advance, it's normal to experience a decrease in hair thickness, luster, and sheen. Especially after age sixty blood circulation becomes less efficient, follicles begin to atrophy, and lubricating oil glands on the scalp don't work as well as they used to.

Naturally fragile older hair is also often the victim of too-vigorous hair-improvement regimens that break off what hasn't already fallen out.

2. *What color are your eyes?* Light-colored eyes usually go with finer-textured hair. And fine hair is subject to many more difficulties than coarse and normal varieties. Whether or not it's light-colored, fine hair is much more liable to damage from chemical waving and coloring treatments and from sun, wind, and other environmental factors. So the point of this question is to make you aware of a possible genetic predisposition to fragile and sensitive hair.

3. *What is your race?* Black people are naturally predisposed to several specific hair problems. For example, many black people who straighten their hair with hot combs are not aware of hot-comb alopecia. This is a case of hair loss caused by overheated pressing oils getting into and killing the hair follicles. Also, certain scalp problems can stem from the predisposition of black skin to form thick keloid scars. And the widespread popularity of Afro styling picks has led to an epidemic of fractured- and breaking-hair problems, as well as traction alopecia (hair loss caused by hair literally being yanked out).

4. *What is the quality of your parents' hair?* Hair quality is a matter of genetic inheritance. The best clue to that inheritance is to take a good look at your parents. It's true that hair traits sometimes skip a generation, but that's not a rule you can depend on. There is a high probability that your hair—and your hair problems—will be similar to those experienced by your parents. If this gives you cause to despair, well, just remember that many things that were hopeless thirty years ago (or whenever your parents were your age) are improvable today.

5. *How much do you brush your hair?* Twenty-five strokes per day is considered optimal for best distribution of natural hair oils. More than that can—and probably

will—cause traction alopecia. You should never use a brush or comb with sharp bristles or teeth, lest they fracture the hair.

6. *How many hairs do you lose per day?* Except for the autumn, when hair loss mysteriously but naturally tends to increase, you should expect to lose between 100 to 200 hairs per day. The unavoidably tedious way to check this is to run a test over any given five-day period. Save all the hairs that collect in your brush or in the shower drain, count them, and take an average. If you lose 1,000 hairs or less over the five days, then you're normal and have no need to worry. If you're losing more, then you've got a problem that's either medical or genetic.

7. *Is your hair normal, oily, or dry?* Remember that if your hair is giving you no problems, leave it alone, don't worry about its being too anything. Dry, flyaway hair is easy enough to recognize, but here's a simple test to determine whether or not your hair is too oily. Wash your hair in the morning and go through a normal day. At six P.M. take a piece of brown paper of the type used for grocery bags, rub it well into the hair on the side of your head, and examine it. You should expect to see some discoloration from natural hair oils, but if the paper becomes translucent, your hair is too oily. If this doesn't bother you, fine. If it does, then adjust your shampoo regimen accordingly.

8. *How often do you shampoo?* Two or three times per week is the optimal average. But oily hair needs more, and dry hair needs less. Make sure your shampoo practices and products match your kind of hair. And remember that shampooing is in no way connected to hair loss.

9. *Do you think your hair grows rapidly, slowly, or at a normal rate?* Some people are fearful that their hair "just doesn't grow." These people often have nothing more serious than slow-growing hair. The normal rate is only .37 millimeters per day, and that isn't fast. As long as your hair isn't

falling out in unusual amounts, slow growth is nothing to be concerned about.

10. *How long is your hair?* Long hair is old hair, and old hair is subject to all sorts of problems that are treatable or at least nothing to be upset about. If you like your hair long, be prepared for inevitable split ends and lack of sheen. Don't worry about it, just trim off the broken ends and use a good conditioner.

11. *What is the climate where you live?* If you make your home in the hot, dry desert, then chances are you'll need extra conditioners to keep your hair looking lustrous. If you live in soggy London, then you'll need extra-strong setting preparations to hold a style. The point here is to consider your environment at the same time you consider your hair problems. Environment plays a major role, and if it can't be modified—for instance, by setting out tubs of water to humidify dry interiors—then you should stick with hairstyles that don't fight it.

12. *What is the physical environment like where you work?* Living in a normal, temperate climate won't help your hair if you spend the whole day in a sealed, dehumidified glass office building or teach for hours under the glaring sun on a tennis court. Again, your problems may be caused by your environment, not by your hair.

13. *Are you active in sports?* Lots of showering, sitting in saunas or steam rooms, lying in the sun, and frolicking on saltwater beaches or in chlorinated pools can all contribute to dry-hair problems.

14. *Are you often in a nervous state?* Stress is your hair's worst enemy. It can easily disrupt your hormonal balance and ruin your hair.

15. *What is the state of your health?* Remember that the hair reflects illnesses about two to three months after they occur. Suddenly bad-looking hair is often a case of delayed noticeable reaction. If your health has improved, and you've

gotten over whatever it was, you should expect the hair to return to normal in another two to three months.

16. *Are you taking any medications?* Certain common pills—such as those for thyroid conditions, diet, water loss, birth control, as well as aspirin and certain multiple vitamins—can wreak havoc on the hair. Every single pill that goes into your mouth, no matter how commonplace, is a medicine. Remember to consider its effect.

17. *How would you describe your diet?* A good diet is one that maintains homeostasis, or the normal status quo. Diets that are too calorie-restrictive can lead to dull, lusterless hair because these diets lack nutrients needed by both follicles and oil glands. Certain bizarre diets can even make the hair fall out.

18. *Are you pregnant or have you just had a baby?* Being pregnant affects your whole body, including your hair. Two to three months after childbirth it is customary for women to experience a fairly massive hair loss, or telogen effluvium, because the trauma at birth tends to throw a disproportionate number of hair follicles into the telogen phase. The effluvium is actually a positive sign, since it means the follicles are again embarking on an anagen growth phase, and new growth is pushing the old telogen hairs out of the follicles. So don't worry.

19. *Are your menstrual periods regular?* If they aren't, it could be a symptom of some hormonal imbalance that may well be affecting your hair as well.

20. *Do you blow dry your hair?* Too much—for example, every day—can dry the hair out and make it susceptible to breakage and unmanageability.

21. *Do you color your hair?* Hair can take only so much coloring. To do it more than twice a month is to risk loss of sheen and highlights; unnatural color and brittleness result as well.

22. *How much time do you spend on your hair?* Some people clearly have trouble taking care of certain hairstyles

because they have no time to do a good job. Constant beauty-parlor visits are not the answer. A large part of looking well groomed depends on choosing a style that fits conveniently into your daily routine.

Part II. The Physical Examination

What follows is a six-part home examination to be performed after you've completed the questionnaire in Part I. Since it's sometimes hard to be really objective with yourself, I'd recommend that you do this examination with a friend.

SECTION 1. EXAMINATION FOR EXCESS BODY HAIR

Take off your clothes, stand in front of a mirror, and observe your skin from head to toe. You may have excess body hair on the face, arms, legs, thighs, anywhere. This is a case when an honest second opinion from a friend can be most helpful. Except in relatively uncommon medical instances, an acceptable amount of body hair is purely a matter of personal taste. And if your body hair bothers neither you nor your intimate loved ones, then put your clothes back on and move to Section 2. If you want to rid yourself of that extra hair, I refer you to Chapter 8, "Away with Body and Facial Hair."

SECTION 2. TESTING HAIR STRENGTH

This test identifies easily fractured hair. With one hand, grasp a swatch of hair with the thickness to your thumb close to the scalp and hold it still. With the other hand twist your anchored swatch between the thumb and first two fingers. Normally nothing should happen. But if hairs break off easily, it's usually an indication of overtreatment with hair chemicals or a particularly bad diet. Easily fractured hair needs a complete holiday from all hair treatments and is usually a sign that it's time to go to a doctor.

SECTION 3. CONFIRMING NORMAL GROWTH-AND-SHED RATIO

This test will tell you whether the anagen (growth cycle) and telogen (shed cycle) hairs on your head are in the proper proportion to one another. If you have good eyesight, you probably won't absolutely need a magnifying glass, but it does help to have one.

The first step is to pluck at least twenty-five of your hairs. Remember you aren't hurting your follicles by doing this, and if you can comfortably pluck more than twenty-five, say, thirty-five or forty, then so much the better. The easiest way to pluck these hairs is to have your friend select groups of four or five hairs, wrap them around the forefinger, and yank quickly and firmly. Take the hairs from different, easily covered locations, and don't worry about bald spots. Most doctors pluck ten hairs at a time with no bad effect.

The anagen to telogen ratio on a normal scalp is approximately 9 to 1. This is to say that it is normal to have nine growing anagen hairs for every telogen hair that's just resting and waiting to fall out. A telogen hair has a little whitish bulb at its base. Some people erroneously think this bulb is some sort of root, but of course you know this isn't so. By contrast, plucked anagen hairs do not have this characteristic bulb at the base.

The anagen-telogen ratio for the eyebrows happens to be exactly the opposite of the one for scalp hair. There are nine telogen eyebrow hairs for every one anagen. Since the telltale telogen bulbs are identical on eyebrow and scalp hairs, it may well be helpful to pluck a few eyebrow hairs first so as to get a readily recognizable telogen hair for comparison's sake.

Take your twenty-five or more scalp hairs, examine each, and sort them. You should have eight or nine anagens for every one telogen. If you don't, your ratio is off and something's wrong. Naturally, you shouldn't do this test in the fall or shortly after childbirth or any traumatic shock or illness. (By the way, save your sample hairs for Section 4.)

SECTION 4. FLAKES AND PROBLEMS ON THE HAIR SHAFT

First you'll want to search for dandruff. You can do this by parting the hair and having your friend-helper look for flakes, then drag your fingernail across the top of the scalp. If either of these tests turns up flakes, heed the warning and get rid of them before the dandruff becomes bad. Dandruff shampoos, sometimes combined with sunlamps and/or sun exposure, are usually all you need to control completely all but the most recalcitrant dandruff.

Next, take those hairs you saved from Section 3, select several likely ones, and examine the length of each with your magnifying glass. The shaft of a normal hair should have a smooth surface and an even diameter. If there are flakes at the base of the hair, it's an indication of dandruff. Little white bumps along the middle of the shaft are often caused by infestations of nits. Split ends that make hair look dull and flyaway can be easily seen under the glass, as can dulling buildups of shampoo or hair-spray residue. You may also discover beads or other genetic irregularities that may give your hair a less than lustrous appearance. Take note of what you see, and plan corrective regimens appropriately.

SECTION 5. CHECKING FOR SIGNS OF HAIR LOSS

You have to lose more than 10 percent of your hair for the loss to become noticeable. There are two simple examination techniques I want you to use in this section. First, without parting the hair, have your assistant observe your head and see if he or she can see through to the scalp. If so, you've probably passed the 10 percent limit. If the noticeable thinning is on the crown and the temples, chances are it's male pattern baldness. If it's on the sides, it may be caused by hot-comb or traction alopecia. And if it's on one spot, it may be a case of fungus infection or alopecia areata.

The other test is to take a swatch of hair on any portion of the scalp and give it a tug. Except for a possible telogen hair or two, normal hair will not come out readily when tugged in this manner. If thirty hairs come out, it's a sign of hair loss from some source—be it medical, psychological, or genetic.

SECTION 6. PREDICTING YOUR
OWN FUTURE APPEARANCE

As long as your anagen-telogen ratio is a normal 9 to 1, you'll continue to look much as you do right now. You can keep tabs on your ratio by doing the test in Section 3 twice a year, say on July Fourth and Christmas.

Looking into the future is chancy at best, but the overwhelming probabilities have it that you will age in patterns similar to those of your parents. Of course this isn't always true, but statistically it's a good bet. Look at pictures of your folks when they were your age and compare them to their present appearance. Your body is probably going to travel a similar path.

Part VI
Formulary

This product formulary is an alphabetical guide to every product in the book. It is not, however, a catalogue of every product on the market. There are eighteen sections, each corresponding to a chapter. A brief description follows every product name; home remedies and household cures are not included.

Chapter 1. Why Hair Grows
None recommended

Chapter 2. Types of Hair and Typical Hair Problems
Alberto VO5—an oily conditioner in a tube, good for dryness
Neutrogena—a mild, pure soap, good for oiliness

Chapter 3. Shampooing
Alberto VO5—well-known product line whose shampoo is good for dry hair
Breck—a reasonably priced shampoo especially good for tinted hair
Bright Side—a shampoo that adds highlights to dull and/or gray hair

Caress—a mild soap containing an oil additive
Clairol Great Body—protein-enriched shampoo for limp hair
Conti—a reasonably priced shampoo with lanolin and olive oil; especially good for dry hair
Dove—a mild soap containing cold-cream additives
Earth Born—an effective and pleasant-smelling shampoo
Fitch—a strong degreasing shampoo
Ivory—a mild soap
Johnson's Baby Shampoo—very mild shampoo
Minipoo—spray-powder dry shampoo that absorbs oil and is brushed out without water
Neutrogena—a mild soap
Pantene—body-building shampoo that contains protein
Prell—a reasonably priced shampoo with excellent lather
Psssst—spray-powder dry shampoo that absorbs oil and is brushed out without water
Purpose—a very mild hypoallergenic shampoo
Revlon Milk Plus 6—body-building protein shampoo
Soap Shampoo—made from plain soap
Toni's Lemon-Up—degreasing shampoo with pleasant lemon scent

Chapter 4. Conditioning

Alberto VO5—this house makes a hot-oil deep conditioner that is applied before the shampoo
Borghese Herbal Blend Conditioning Hair Pack—pleasant-smelling, shine-inducing conditioner
Braggi Hair and Scalp Conditioner—just as good a conditioner for women as it is for men
Buttermilk by Clairol—acid conditioner good for adding sheen
Clairol Conditioner Beauty Pack—conditioner for problem damaged hair
Elizabeth Arden's Especially Effective Hair Conditioner—a good lotion conditioner

Hair Care Problem Solver—Helena Rubinstein's shampoo containing soluble beads of conditioner

Long and Silky—Clairol's fast-acting acid conditioner for very long hair

L'Oréal's Oleocap—a do-it-yourself home hot-oil conditioner kit, good for damaged hair

Maintain—a deluxe lotion conditioner

Palm Beach Firm and Fill—a protein superconditioner used on head wrapped with a moist hot towel

Phinal Phase by Redken—reasonably priced acid cream rinse that adds sheen

Skin Dew—Helena Rubinstein's no-rinse postshampoo conditioning additive

Unicure—very acid conditioner

Vidal Sassoon's Protein Cream Hair Remoisturizer—protein-coating conditioner

Chapter 5. Blow Dryers

Blow-care by Cosmetco—a protective conditioner applied before blow drying

Clairol AB-1, AB-2—recommended blow dryers

GE SD-1, SD-2, STC1, Zoom 'n Groom—recommended blow dryers

Gillette THD2, THD2A—recommended blow dryers

Hamilton Beach 423—recommended blow dryer

The Heat Solution by Pantene—a protein protective conditioner applied to hair before blow drying

Kindness—Clairol's spray protective conditioner applied to hair before blow drying

Lady Schick 338, Speed Styler 352—recommended dryers

Norelco Shape 'n Dry 750—recommended blow dryer

Northern 1800—recommended blow dryer

Panasonic EH-741, EH-745—recommended blow dryers

Remington HW-3, HW-6, 600—recommended blow dryers

Schick 336—recommended blow dryer

Sunbeam EC-5, EC-6—recommended blow dryers
Zap by Clairol—protective protein conditioner applied to hair before blow drying

Chapter 6. Home Styling and Grooming
Alberto VO5—dressing for dull and dry hair
Alberto VO5 Hair Spray—holding hair spray
Allercreme—hypoallergenic hair spray
Aquaphore—made for skin but can be used for dry hair
Breck—a holding hair spray
Brillcreem—dressing for dry hair
Clairol Electric Rollers—electrically heated quick-hair-setting kit
Clairol Final Net—holding hair spray
Crazy Curl by Clairol—recommended curling iron
Drest—greaseless dressing for normal hair
GE Electric Rollers—electrically heated quick-hair-setting kit
Gillette's Dry Look—holding hair spray
Groom 'n Clean—greaseless dressing for normal hair
Hair Spray de Pantene—hair spray with protein
Lady Schick Quick Curls—a recommended curling iron
L'Oréal's Elnett—holding hair spray
Marcelle—hypoallergenic hair spray
Oster Mist Set—recommended curling iron
Pantene—protein-based hair body builder
Pinot—greaseless dressing for normal to oily hair
Protein 29—hair spray with protein
Redken—hair spray with protein
Score—very greaseless dressing for normal hair
Self Styling Adorn—a holding hair spray
Thickit—protein-based hair body builder
Vaseline—made for skin but can be useful on dry hair
Vitalis—greaseless dressing good for normal to oily hair
Vitapointe by Clairol—dressing for dull and dry hair, less greasy than Alberto VO5
Wildroot—dressing for dry hair

Chapter 7. Hair Care for Black People
Afro Sheen Hair Spray—oil conditioner in spray-can form
Apex—a pressing oil used with a hot comb
Betadine—an antibiotic shampoo
Dax—a pomade
Dixie Peach—a pomade
Duke—a pomade
Gloss—pressing oil used with a hot comb
Posner Pressing Oil Glossine—pressing oil used with a hot comb
Tetracycline—prescription antibiotic often prescribed for pseudofolliculitis
Ultra Sheen Conditioner and Hair Dress—a pomade
Vaseline—meant for skin but good for dull hair in small amounts
Vitapointe—a grooming oil

Chapter 8. Away with Body and Facial Hair
Aimé—a bleaching cream
Bu-To—cream depilatory
Jolen—a bleaching cream
Nair—cream depilatory
Neet—cream depilatory
Noxzema—a soothing shaving cream
Nudit—cream depilatory
Perma-Tweez—battery-operated home epilator
Shimmy Shins—cream depilatory
Sleek—cream depilatory
Surgex—cream depilatory
Williams 'Lectric Shave—preshave lotion for electric razors
Zip Depilatory—home wax hair remover

Chapter 9. Hair Coloring
Blond Silk by Revlon—a toner to soften harsh hair coloring that sometimes comes from peroxide

Born Blond Lightener by Clairol—peroxide bleach with conditioner

Born Blond Lotion Toner by Clairol—a toner to soften harsh hair color that sometimes comes from peroxide

Breck Hair Color—full line of hair dyes

Clairol Balsam Color—full line of hair dyes

Clairol's Clairoxide—hydrogen-peroxide bleaching solution

Clairol's Frost and Tip—hair-painting kit

Clairol's Nice 'n Easy—full line of packaged home hair-coloring kits

Color Silk by Revlon—full line of hair dyes

Come Alive Grey by Clairol—temporary hair dye without peroxide

Delete by Roux—color dye solvent

Effasol by L'Oréal—color dye solvent

European Naturals by Alberto Culver—full line of hair dyes

Excellence Extra Rich Hair Color by L'Oréal—full line of hair dyes

Fanci-Full by Roux—temporary-hair-dye line without peroxide

Fanci-Tone by Roux—a full line of hair dyes

Happiness by Clairol—semipermanent hair dye without peroxide

Henna—organic plant-derived red dye

Hydrogen peroxide—a basic hair bleach incorporated in many other products but also effective by itself

Lady Grecian Formula—metallic-dye hair restorer without peroxide

Lemon Go Lightly by Clairol—peroxide bleach with conditioner

L'Oréal's Preference—full line of packaged home hair-coloring kits

L'Oréal Preference Perfect Blond—a toner to soften harsh hair color that sometimes comes from peroxide

Loving Care Color Foam by Clairol—semipermanent hair dye without peroxide

Loving Care Hair Color Lotion by Clairol—semipermanent hair dye without peroxide

Metalex by Clairol—color dye solvent

Midnight Sun by Clairol—gentle peroxide lightener to use in the sun

Miss Clairol Hair Color Bath Creme Formula—full line of hair dyes

Nestlé Protein Color Rinse—temporary hair dye without peroxide

Nice 'n Easy by Clairol—full line of hair dyes

Noreen Color Hair Rinse—temporary hair dye without peroxide

Picture Perfect Color Rinse by Clairol—temporary hair dye without peroxide

Preference by L'Oréal—full line of hair dyes

Quiet Touch Hair Painting Kit—hair-painting kit

RD—metallic-dye hair restorer without peroxide

Remov-zit by Clairol—color dye solvent

Revlon's Color Silk Crystal Lights—a toner to soften harsh hair color that sometimes comes from peroxide

Silk and Silver Color Lotion—semipermanent hair dye without peroxide

Snow Silk Lightener by Revlon—peroxide bleach with conditioner

Streaks 'n Tips by Nestlé—temporary hair dye without peroxide

Summer Blond by Clairol—peroxide bleach with conditioner

Summer Blond Hair Painting Kit—hair-painting kit

Sun-In by Gillette—a gentle peroxide lightener to use in the sun

Touch of Silver by L'Oréal—semipermanent hair dye without peroxide

Tried and True by Max Factor—full line of hair dyes
Ultra Silk Hair Lightener by Revlon—peroxide bleach with conditioner
Young Blond by L'Oréal—gentle peroxide lightener to use in the sun
Youthair—metallic-dye hair restorer without peroxide

Chapter 10. Waving and Straightening
Amino Organic Permanent Wave—home hair.permanent kit
Apex Natural Perm—a sodium-hydroxide home hair straightener
Bobbi—home hair-permanent kit
Clairol Condition—a postpermanent curl relaxer
Curl-Away by Continental Labs—thioglycolate home hair straightener
Curlaxer by Posner—sodium-bisulfite home hair straightener
Curl Free by Gillette—sodium-bisulfite home hair straightener
Curls Away by Richard Hudnut—thioglycolate home hair straightener
Ever Perm by Helene Curtis—sodium-hydroxide home hair straightener
Go Straight by Nutritonic—thioglycolate home hair straightener
Hair Strate by Summit Labs—sodium-hydroxide home hair straightener
Metalex Conditioner and Corrective—a postpermanent curl relaxer
Royal Crown Relaxer Permanent—sodium-hydroxide home hair straightener
Set Me Straight by Rexall—thioglycolate home hair straightener
Smooth Away by Helene Curtis—thioglycolate home hair straightener

Straight Set by Max Factor—thioglycolate home hair straightener

Sudden Silk by Evans—thioglycolate home hair straightener

Super Toni by Gillette—home hair-permanent kit

Twin Conditioning Gentle Toni by Gillette—home hair-permanent kit

Ultra-Wave by Johnson—sodium-hydroxide home hair straightener

U.N.C.U.R.L. by Clairol—sodium-bisulfite home hair straightener

Vege-Kurl—sodium-bisulfite home hair straightener

Wellastrate by Wella—thioglycolate home hair straightener

Chapter 11. Hairstyles and Professional Stylists
None recommended

Chapter 12. Hair-Treatment Salons and Studios:
Do They Really Work?
None recommended

Chapter 13. Diseases of the Hair and What
the Doctor Can Do
Betadine—antibacterial shampoo

Enden—OTC dandruff shampoo

Griseofulvin—strong prescription antifungal medicine in pill form

Head 'n Shoulders—OTC dandruff shampoo

Kwell—prescription lotion and shampoo for nit or lice infestation

P and S Solution—medicine for psoriasis of the scalp

Sebulex—OTC dandruff shampoo

Selsun—OTC dandruff shampoo

Tinactin—medicine in cream, liquid, and powder form for fungal infections

Vanseb T—OTC dandruff shampoo
Zetar—OTC dandruff shampoo
Zinc Oxide—a soothing paste for eczematous irritations
Zincon—OTC dandruff shampoo

Chapter 14. Nutrition and Your Hair
Recommended Books:
The Brand Name Calorie Counter, edited by Corinne
　　Netzer, published by Dell
The Dictionary of Calories and Carbohydrates, edited by
　　Barbara Kraus, published by New American Library

Chapter 15. The Medical Causes of Hair Loss
Iron pills—for treating mild iron deficiency
Premarin—prescription estrogen in pill or lotion form

Chapter 16. Calm Down and Grow Hair
Valium—a safe prescription tranquilizer

Chapter 17. Hair Replacement
None recommended

Chapter 18. The Do-It-Yourself Home Hair Analysis
None recommended

Index